The Acquisition of Drugs and Biologics for Chemical and Biological Warfare Defense

Department of Defense Interactions with the Food and Drug Administration

Richard A. Rettig
Jennifer Brower
with Orlie Yaniv

Prepared for the Office of the Secretary of Defense

National Defense Research Institute | RAND Health

RAND

Approved for public release; distribution unlimited

The research described in this report was sponsored by the Office of the Secretary of Defense (OSD). The research was conducted jointly by RAND Health's Center for Military Health Policy Research and the Forces and Resources Policy Center of the National Defense Research Institute, a federally funded research and development center supported by the OSD, the Joint Staff, the unified commands, and the defense agencies under Contract DASW01-01-C-0004.

Library of Congress Cataloging-in-Publication Data

Rettig, Richard A.
The acquisition of drug and biologics for chemical and biological warfare defense : Department of Defense interactions with the Food and Drug Administration / Richard A. Rettig, Jennifer Brower, with Orlie Yaniv.
p. cm.
"MR-1659."
Includes bibliographical references and index.
ISBN 0-8330-3450-2 (pbk.)
1. Chemical agents (Munitions)—Safety measures. 2. Biological weapons—Safety measures. 3. United States—Armed Forces—Medical supplies. 4. United States. Dept. of Defense—Procurement. 5. United States. Food and Drug Administration. I. Brower, Jennifer, 1967– II. Yaniv, Orlie. III.Title.

UG447.R4597 2003
358'.34'0973—dc22

2003015371

RAND is a nonprofit institution that helps improve policy and decisionmaking through research and analysis. RAND® is a registered trademark. RAND's publications do not necessarily reflect the opinions or policies of its research sponsors.

Published 2003 by RAND
1700 Main Street, P.O. Box 2138, Santa Monica, CA 90407-2138
1200 South Hayes Street, Arlington, VA 22202-5050
201 North Craig Street, Suite 202, Pittsburgh, PA 15213-1516
RAND URL: http://www.rand.org/
To order RAND documents or to obtain additional information, contact Distribution Services: Telephone: (310) 451-7002; Fax: (310) 451-6915; Email: order@rand.org

PREFACE

In fulfilling the national security objective of the acquisition of drugs and biologics for chemical and biological warfare (CBW) defense, the U.S. Department of Defense (DoD) depends in part on the independent judgment and decisions of another federal government agency, the U.S. Food and Drug Administration (FDA). FDA, exercising authority under the Federal Food, Drug, and Cosmetic Act and the Public Health Service Act, and the implementing regulations of these statutes, regulates the testing of drugs for safety and effectiveness in all stages of development. The agency prescribes the manufacturing standards that must be met before products can be released for human use.

DoD's dependence on FDA has been brought into focus in the past decade—initially by the experience of the 1990–1991 Gulf War and more recently by the difficulties of obtaining enough licensed anthrax vaccine to immunize all military personnel. However, these events are but the immediate manifestation of a continuing dependent relationship that involves three types of interactions: licensing CBW drugs and biologics, especially vaccines; using Investigational New Drugs in military combat (and other special situations); and ensuring the compliance of producers with manufacturing requirements.

DoD has not been well organized to respond to FDA. This report proposes various education and training programs that should be initiated for all defense personnel engaged in the development or acquisition of drugs and biologics for CBW defense. It also recommends organizational changes in the Office of the Secretary of

Defense (OSD) to centralize the authority for interactions between DoD and FDA.

This research will interest DoD policymakers involved in research and development, acquisition, and medical use policy related to defense against CBW agents; producers of drugs and vaccines for military use, especially for CBW defense; FDA officials whose responsibilities have been reordered by the events of September 11, 2001; officials in the Department of Health and Human Services and in the Department of Homeland Security; and the interested public.

This research was sponsored by the Deputy Assistant to the Secretary of Defense for Chemical and Biological Defense and was carried out jointly by RAND's Center for Military Health Policy Research and the Acquisition and Technology Policy Center of the National Defense Research Institute. The latter is a federally funded research and development center sponsored by OSD, the Joint Staff, the unified commands, and the defense agencies in the fulfillment of national security objectives involving the development and acquisition of drugs and biologics, mostly vaccines, for CBW defense.

CONTENTS

Preface iii

Executive Summary vii

Acknowledgments xvii

Abbreviations xix

Chapter One
INTRODUCTION 1
A Matter of Perspective 3
Background 4
Organization of the Report 7
Research Methods 8

Chapter Two
THE CHALLENGES OF ACQUISITION 11
Licensing 12
The Department of Defense's Organization for FDA Interaction 16
Using Investigational New Drugs 19
Manufacturing 23
The Three-Way Relationship 30
CBER Team Biologics 33

Chapter Three
THE INDUSTRIAL MODEL 37
The High-Control Industrial Model 37
Education and Training 41
Regulatory Affairs: A Corporate Function 43

Chapter Four
SUMMARY AND RECOMMENDATIONS 47
No Change 49
Education and Training 49
Organizational Change 55
Conclusion 59

Appendix
PRIVATE PROVIDERS OF FDA-RELATED EDUCATION AND TRAINING 61

Interviews 65

References 71

About the Authors 77

EXECUTIVE SUMMARY

Chemical and biological threats confront U.S. military personnel today both overseas and in the continental United States, whether in defensive, peacekeeping, or offensive situations. Defenses against such threats are both medical and nonmedical. Drugs and biologics, mainly vaccines, constitute the primary medical defenses. Consequently, efforts of the U.S. Department of Defense (DoD) to protect American troops require the acquisition of drugs and biologics for chemical and biological warfare (CBW) defense. The objective of this acquisition, as is the case for other acquisitions, is to obtain the desired supply of a given product at an acceptable price.

This study includes both drugs and biologics, but it emphasizes the latter (mainly focusing on vaccines, a subset of biologics). Vaccines provide advanced protection against biological warfare threats via immunization of at-risk troops—and prior protection is a high priority within DoD. In contrast, drugs are useful mainly in treating already-exposed troops. Vaccine development is also more complicated than drug development because it typically involves manipulating live organisms, whereas drugs consist of more-stable chemical entities.

DoD has two distinct roles during the acquisition of drugs and biologics for CBW defense: purchaser and developer. As *purchaser* of a drug approved by the U.S. Food and Drug Administration (FDA) for which a commercial market exists, DoD simply buys what it needs at the market price; DoD acquisition of influenza vaccine is a good example of this. However, when the market is limited mainly to military use, even for a drug that is approved by FDA, DoD's role as purchaser becomes more complicated. An example of this is the acquisition of adenovirus vaccine for preventing upper respiratory disease among military trainees. DoD's providing of an inadequate market resulted in the sole manufacturer ceasing its production (Committee on a Strategy for Minimizing the Impact . . . , 2000).

DoD is not just another purchaser in a commercial market, however. It becomes a *developer* of drugs when demand is mainly or exclusively for military use. Under these circumstances, DoD requirements for CBW defense drugs involve the department in the full spectrum of research, development, testing for safety and effectiveness through clinical trials or alternate means, production, acquisition, and issues of medical use. (This may also be the case for naturally occurring diseases that rarely appear in the United States and for which the domestic civilian market is limited.)

In the same way that all roads led to Rome in the ancient world, all issues related to drug and biologic development lead to and through FDA. The agency regulates all aspects of vaccine and pharmaceutical research, development, production, marketing, and use. As a result, DoD encounters FDA in all aspects of procuring CBW pharmaceuticals. Successful DoD acquisition of CBW drugs and vaccines depends in large measure on DoD's understanding of the regulatory requirements of FDA and on incorporating this knowledge into its own policies, organization, budgets, and procedures. However, because DoD has not viewed acquisition of CBW drugs as a primary mission, its understanding of FDA has often been lacking, especially at the highest levels of the department. Adequate attention to FDA is essential for DoD to fulfill its national security objectives related to CBW pharmaceuticals. To acquire adequate supplies of CBW drugs and vaccines at a reasonable price, it is essential that DoD establish and maintain ongoing and productive relationships with FDA at both policy and operations levels.

Acquisition involves three major interactions between DoD and FDA related to CBW defense: (1) licensing of new CBW drugs by FDA; (2) use of Investigational New Drugs (INDs) in combat; and (3) manufacturing of drugs and vaccines. Licensing by FDA of new pharmaceuticals is critical to the fulfillment of DoD objectives for CBW defense. The DoD investment in research and development for pharmaceuticals of military interest primarily is a necessary but not sufficient way to obtain licensed products. The DoD acquisition objective requires that products receive FDA licensing.

Closely linked to licensing are the interactions related to the use of INDs in combat (and other special) situations in which the threat of enemy use of chemical and/or biological agents is genuine. However, many CBW drugs and biologics in the DoD pipeline never move beyond the IND stage, largely because few economic incentives exist for pharmaceutical firms to develop military use–only products and because of the difficulty of generating data on efficacy. Therefore, DoD must understand the consequences that follow if pharmaceuticals languish in the IND phase.

Three factors—ease of use, recordkeeping, and acceptance by military personnel and the wider public—underline the importance of licensed drugs. By contrast, the regulatory requirements of IND use, the burden of recordkeeping, and the limited public acceptance (and even rejection) highlight their limits:

- Licensed drugs are *easy to use*. Decisions to use them are medical decisions, made by field commanders acting on the advice of their field surgeons, and they are administered by medical personnel. INDs, however, are far more difficult to use: They may be used under all the restrictions of IND use, including informed consent, which are difficult to meet in wartime; or, in rarer situations, informed consent can be waived—but only by the President of the United States (and even then many IND-related restrictions apply) (Rettig, 1999, pp. 97–99).
- *Recordkeeping* for the use of licensed drugs is a routine part of medical care of deployed troops. By contrast, recordkeeping requirements for IND use are substantial. Failure to comply with FDA requirements for keeping adequate records characterized the use of INDs in the Gulf War, as it did in the use of the tick-borne encephalitis vaccine in Bosnia.
- Finally, *military and public acceptance* during and after conflict is influenced strongly by whether a drug is licensed or whether it is classified as an IND. An IND for CBW defense may be the best available treatment in the face of a lethal chemical or biological threat, and the risk-benefit calculus must include the risk of nonuse in the face of such a threat. Although an IND may be

> described technically or legally as "not yet approved" by FDA, the connotation of "investigational" as meaning "experimental" cannot be escaped—nor can the negative effect of taking an "investigational" drug on troop acceptance during a conflict. Importantly, public and political criticism afterward cannot be avoided.

Because of these factors, DoD acquisition should aim to increase the number of licensed products and, in so doing, reduce the department's reliance on INDs.

The third interaction between DoD and FDA involves the manufacturing of drugs and biologics. FDA has markedly increased scrutiny of manufacturing of both biological and pharmaceutical products in recent years. The difficulties of obtaining anthrax vaccine, an FDA-licensed product, from BioPort, the sole manufacturer of the vaccine, were primarily manufacturing problems. DoD, the primary customer of BioPort, had significant leverage over the manufacturer because of its contract for anthrax vaccine. But the department failed to anticipate the engagement of FDA and its regulations during and after the refurbishing of the production facility. Beyond the anthrax vaccine experience, however, FDA's Center for Biologic Evaluation and Research has increased its scrutiny of all biologic manufacturing in recent years, partly because of technological advances in measuring purity of biologic products. In addition, the agency's Center for Drug Evaluation and Research has also increased its attention to manufacturing compliance by regulated pharmaceutical firms. As a result, in its relationship with FDA, DoD's acquisition of pharmaceuticals must in part focus on manufacturing issues.

The ability of DoD to obtain the drugs needed for CBW defense is influenced by a number of factors, of which DoD-FDA relations are only one. The lack of economic incentives for commercial pharmaceutical firms to produce drugs and biologics for military use and the appropriate departmental organization for vaccine acquisition are broader contextual issues. In general, pharmaceutical firms have less reason to develop vaccines than drugs: Vaccines provide less than 10 percent of pharmaceutical industry revenues. For drugs and vaccines intended mainly for military use, the market is simply too small to interest private-sector investment in bringing such products through FDA licensing. Furthermore, the vaccine industry, as distinct from the pharmaceutical industry of which it is a part, is small and unstable: It consists of four major pharmaceutical firms (Merck, Aventis Pasteur, Glaxo, and Wyeth), a number of smaller legacy manufacturers that produce vaccines licensed in an earlier era (e.g., BioPort), and a larger number of more-recent biotech firms (e.g., MedImmune). Although biotech firms have been the source of many promising ideas, most have yet to bring products through the FDA regulatory process to the market. Finally, the costs of developing a new drug are very high. Estimates by the Tufts [University] Center for the Study of Drug Development updated the $287 million estimate of 1987 to $802 million in 2002. An expert panel convened by DoD estimated development costs at $300–400 million per vaccine. Although these estimates are widely known in the pharmaceutical industry, DoD budgets have not reflected them.

Organizationally, several offices within DoD are responsible for various aspects of drug and vaccine development and acquisition. For more than a decade, the need for a government-owned, contractor-operated (GOCO) facility for vaccine production has been debated as a way to offset DoD's inability to produce licensed CBW drugs and the limited private-sector incentives to manufacture these products. The independent panel of experts, known as the Vaccine Study Panel, that advised DoD in 2001 on vaccine manufacturing issues basically endorsed the GOCO argument. In addition, the Gilmore Commission[1] and the Institute of Medicine have recommended a GOCO, or its equivalent, relative to national vaccine needs for national and homeland security. These broader organizational issues are important; however, they are beyond the scope of this report.

In this context, DoD interactions with FDA are a critical and often-overlooked issue. DoD responsibility for CBW drug and biologics development is distributed across several organizations within the department. The Chemical and Biological Defense Program, which includes separate programs for chemical and biological defense, oversees drug and vaccine development for CBW defense through an Office of the Secretary of Defense (OSD) steering committee. The Deputy Assistant to the Secretary of Defense for Chemical and Bio-

[1]Officially the Advisory Panel to Assess Domestic Response Capabilities for Terrorism Involving Weapons of Mass Destruction.

logical Defense (DATSD[CBD]) provides policy and budgetary oversight to these programs, for which the U.S. Army is the Executive Agent. However, no central OSD authority exists to manage DoD's critical interactions with FDA.

DoD drug and biologics development for CBW defense control is fragmented within the department and between the government and private contractors. DoD acquisition personnel and DoD contractors often lack the technical and managerial expertise and experience for working with FDA. Often, too few resources are allocated to CBW drugs and biologics acquisition. Finally, experience in generating surrogate efficacy data using animal studies for CBW defense drugs that cannot be tested on humans is only now being acquired.

Diffusion of authority and responsibility within DoD characterize the overall management of the biological warfare vaccine development effort in interactions with FDA. During the DoD effort to obtain anthrax vaccine from BioPort, a complicated three-way interaction between DoD, BioPort, and FDA took place. Meetings between BioPort and FDA were attended by as many as 20 to 30 senior DoD officials, both civilian and uniformed, representing half a dozen separate agencies. Many of these people had little education or expertise relevant to FDA. No single organization exercised authority for OSD. This made it significantly more difficult for DoD and FDA to work together with BioPort to resolve outstanding issues.

The industrial model of drug development, including pharmaceutical firm interactions with FDA, contrasts sharply with that of DoD. In general, industry organization for drug development involves a clear corporate strategy of high control. This is especially true for vaccines, as quality control over the manufacture of living organisms (biologics) is substantially harder than for the manufacture of chemical molecules (drugs). Second, industry makes a deep investment in education and training (E&T) of its personnel in manufacturing. At Merck Manufacturing Division, for example, formal training includes those who handle product through middle managers to senior managers, including the president of the division. Finally, the pharmaceutical industry organizes interactions with FDA as a corporate function, reporting independently of product development to the highest levels of the organization. Dealing with FDA is not delegated to subordinate organizations. Moreover, a single point of contact within the pharmaceutical firm coordinates all interactions with FDA for a specific product.

What options does DoD have in addressing the management of its relations with FDA? Three basic options are:

- do nothing to change the current system
- to increase expertise and understanding, establish an E&T program on FDA regulation of drugs and biologics for all department acquisition personnel and others with relevant authority
- introduce organizational changes to coordinate, centralize, and improve DoD-FDA interactions.

The second and third options are not mutually exclusive.

Doing nothing makes little sense given the priority that DoD attaches to acquiring additional CBW drugs and biologics. Given that priority, DoD's dependence on FDA in fulfilling its essential national security objectives means that effective management of the relationship with FDA must also be a high priority. Interestingly, the nation recently faced the prospect of another war with Iraq, and the threat of CBW agents, with only one more licensed drug—pyridostigmine bromide—than it had more than a decade ago during the Gulf War.

The second option, establishing a formal E&T program within DoD for personnel who deal with FDA and its regulatory requirements, is needed. The necessity arises from the dependence of DoD on FDA decisions about drugs, the comprehensive nature of FDA regulation, the continual change in those regulations and in FDA's interpretation of them, and the limited information each agency has about the other. We recommend an E&T program that spans all functions—from research and development through manufacturing and production, acquisition and purchasing, and medical use—involved in the acquisition process and for all personnel, from the operations level through policy. This program should focus on FDA and its regulatory authority, policies, and procedures and the implications of this regulatory regime for DoD. It should be comprehensive. It should compare in quality to similar programs in the pharmaceutical industry and to the E&T that DoD routinely provides in many other areas.

The education program should be required for all personnel involved in the development and acquisition of drugs and biologics for CBW defense, including DoD officials at all levels—policy and operational—regardless of whether their dealings with FDA are continuous or episodic, frequent or infrequent. A limitation of such a program is that high-level acquisition personnel having episodic involvement in the acquisition of CBW drugs and vaccines have many other claims on their time. Typically, the acquisition of pharmaceuticals is secondary for them; they have limited knowledge of and experience with FDA; and they have little interest in training that lacks an immediate benefit. However, as they cannot avoid dealing with FDA in the procurement of drugs and vaccines of unique military interest, their participation is essential. In addition, the constant change of personnel characteristic of DoD means that few people develop long-term expertise in a specific area of pharmaceutical development or FDA regulation of the same. The education program should be pursued regardless of the organizational approach—GOCO or prime contractor—that DoD pursues for CBW defense. The "on the job" training of acquisition personnel about FDA of the past decade was inadequate to the task.

Three sources of FDA E&T programs exist: the private sector, FDA, and DoD. In addition, DoD has the capability of integrating FDA-related material into established defense acquisition curricula. DoD also needs to engage FDA in defining a national security agenda for drug and biologics development because of the increased appreciation of the threat of biological weapons. The CBW threat, both to national and homeland security, raises the question of whether current FDA regulations developed for commercial drug development are adequate to meet new national needs. To this end, DoD and FDA should jointly organize an annual meeting focused on general issues pertaining to CBW defense.

However, an E&T program alone is not a sufficient response to the issues raised by DoD interactions with FDA. The third option, implementing organizational changes, is also required. At present, OSD deals with FDA through the DATSD(CBD) and the Assistant Secretary of Defense for Health Affairs (ASD[HA]). The Joint Vaccine Acquisition Program has a small staff that deals with FDA relations, but it relies mainly on its prime system contractor, the DynPort Vaccine Company, for managing most interactions with FDA. The

Army's Medical Research and Materiel Command relies on its own personnel to deal with FDA in the early stages of research and then transfers that responsibility to contractors (i.e., pharmaceutical firms) in the licensure and production stages.

More fundamentally, the absence of clear departmental authority for dealing with FDA not only risks repeating the anthrax vaccine experience but also inhibits the department from developing a coherent strategy related to interactions with FDA. The department remains vulnerable to high-priority acquisition decisions for CBW drugs and biologics, which invariably involve FDA, being made by acquisition officials with little prior knowledge, experience, or training pertinent to FDA regulatory requirements.

We recommend first that DoD consolidate authority for all its relationships with FDA related to drugs and biologics for CBW defense into a single OSD office. The two candidates for this responsibility are the ASD(HA) and the DATSD(CBD). Health Affairs lacks authority for research and development and acquisition; it is therefore a poor candidate for being the primary OSD point of contact with FDA on acquisition-related issues. The primary FDA-related function of ASD(HA) for CBW defense is to determine the medical indications of use, both for licensed drugs and IND-classified drugs. Therefore, we conclude that Health Affairs should remain the primary OSD authority for this purpose. Moreover, it would encounter an institutional conflict of interest if it were assigned the acquisition function: Having simultaneous responsibility for acquisition would compromise the responsibility for the safety effectiveness of medicines for military personnel.

OSD authority would best be vested in the DATSD(CBD) for determining when and how DoD interacts with FDA for all CBW drugs and vaccines. Centralization of OSD authority for FDA relations is intended to clarify who speaks to FDA, who speaks for the Secretary of Defense, and who answers to Congress on issues of CBW defense. It need not preclude delegation of authority for specific drugs or biologics.

Second, we recommend that the position of Director of Regulatory Affairs be established in DATSD(CBD) to provide a single point of contact for relations with FDA and improve the full cycle of CBW research, development, and manufacturing. This official should

- establish general DoD policy for dealing with FDA for all CBW defense drugs and vaccines
- function as the primary point of contact for all DoD relations with FDA for any specific CBW defense drug or biologic
- delegate operational responsibility for a specific CBW defense drug or vaccine to the appropriate DoD agency
- establish DoD general policy for relations with private contractors engaged by the department in the development of a CBW defense drug or biologic
- ensure the availability of E&T programs related to FDA and the participation of all appropriate personnel in such programs.

We do not recommend the creation of a large, centralized bureaucracy at the OSD level but suggest a single point of contact for coordination with FDA for CBW drugs and biologics.

Third, given the complementarities of vaccine development for biological warfare defense and for infectious diseases, we also recommend that comparable authority for the acquisition of vaccines for infectious diseases be established in OSD.

ACKNOWLEDGMENTS

Many individuals' expertise contributed to our understanding of the complex interagency relationships between DoD and FDA. The substantial number of interviewees listed at the end of this report alone indicates the magnitude of the debt we owe to these individuals. They gave substantial time to meet with us or respond to our telephone inquiries. Our thanks to them are great.

In DoD, Anna Johnson-Winegar, Deputy Assistant Secretary of Defense for Chemical and Biological Defense, requested the study and provided important guidance at critical points. In her office, Robert Borowski provided sustained counsel throughout the study. The DoD interviewees included a number of military and civilian officials, most active and some retired. Our debt to them is substantial.

In FDA, Mark Elengold, Deputy Director, CBER, candidly shared his views on the issues with which we were wrestling. He made CBER professional staff members available to us, and we took great advantage of their insights.

Many individuals in the pharmaceutical industry provided important information about the corporate regulatory affairs function, which helps manage relations with FDA. Thanks go especially to Bruce Burlington of Wyeth; Franklin Top of MedImmune, who chaired the expert panel that advised DoD on vaccines; and John Dingerdissen, then with Merck Vaccines.

Within RAND, Ross Anthony, head of the Military Health Program, provided helpful oversight and guidance. Elisa Eiseman reviewed an early draft of a technical chapter on vaccines and clarified some important questions. Two reviewers of the draft report, Richard A. Merrill of the University of Virginia School of Law and Bernie Rostker of RAND, also contributed to a stronger final report.

We are responsible, of course, for any errors that remain.

ABBREVIATIONS

ASD(HA)	Assistant Secretary of Defense for Health Affairs
AVA	Anthrax Vaccine Absorbed
AVIP	Anthrax Vaccine Immunization Program
BLA	Biologic License Application
BT	botulinum toxoid
CBER	Center for Biologics Evaluation and Research
CBW	chemical and biological warfare
CDER	Center for Drug Evaluation and Research
CDRH	Center for Devices and Radiological Health
CFR	Code of Federal Regulations
cGMP	current Good Manufacturing Practice
DATSD(CBD)	Deputy Assistant to the Secretary of Defense for Chemical and Biological Defense
DIA	Drug Information Association
DoD	U.S. Department of Defense
E&T	education and training
FDA	U.S. Food and Drug Administration

FDLI	Food and Drug Law Institute
FFDCA	Federal Food, Drug, and Cosmetic Act
GCP	Good Clinical Practice
Gilmore Commission	Advisory Panel to Assess Domestic Response Capabilities for Terrorism Involving Weapons of Mass Destruction
GLP	Good Laboratory Practice
GMP	Good Manufacturing Practice
GOCO	government owned, contractor operated
ICAF	Industrial College of the Armed Forces
IND	Investigational New Drug
JPEO-CBD	Joint Program Executive Office for Chemical-Biological Defense
JPO-BD	Joint Program Office for Biological Defense
JVAP	Joint Vaccine Acquisition Program
MBPI	Michigan Biologics Products Institute
NDA	New Drug Application
ORA	Office of Regulatory Affairs
ORO	Office of Regional Operations
OSD	Office of the Secretary of Defense
PB	pyridostigmine bromide
PEO	Program Executive Officer
PHSA	Public Health Service Act
QA	quality assurance
RA	regulatory affairs

RAPS	Regulatory Affairs Professionals Society
USAMRIID	U.S. Army Medical Research Institute of Infectious Diseases
USAMRMC	U.S. Army Medical Research and Materiel Command
VAE	Vaccine Acquisition Executive

Chapter One

INTRODUCTION

National security threats to the United States today include chemical and biological agents. Military personnel face such threats both in the continental United States and overseas, whether in defensive, peacekeeping, or offensive actions. Awareness of military chemical and biological warfare (CBW) threats reemerged forcefully in the Gulf War. The subsequent disclosure of the CBW capabilities of the former Soviet Union, the discovery of an Iraqi CBW capability after the Gulf War, and the recognition that a number of hostile governments have developed or are developing some CBW capability reinforced the danger (Alibek, 2000). The September 11, 2001, terrorist attacks on the World Trade Center and Pentagon further heightened awareness of terrorist threats to the continental United States.[1] The distribution of anthrax through the U.S. Postal System in the months following September 11 reinforced the imminence of the biological warfare threat and made its disruptive effects concrete.

The U.S. government under President Nixon formally renounced any intention to use CBW weapons offensively. However, the United States has continued to devote resources to passive and active defensive measures against such weapons. Passive defenses include enhanced detection of CBW agents, decontamination, and physical protection of individuals and units. Active measures include the medical treatment of exposed individuals, mainly by pharmaceuti-

---

[1]Inglesby, Henderson, et al. (1999); Henderson, Inglesby, et al. (1999); Inglesby, Dennis, et al. (2000); Arnon, Schechter, et al. (2001); Dennis, Inglesby, et al. (2001). See also Gilmore Commission (2001); Weiss (2001), p. A24; and Fialka et al. (2001).

cals (drugs), and the protection of personnel by immunization, mainly by vaccines.

The objective of the U.S. Department of Defense (DoD) in the acquisition of drugs and biologics for CBW defense, or for any other use, is to obtain the desired supply of a given product at an acceptable price. This objective involves DoD in two distinct roles: purchaser and developer.

When the drug or biological in question has been approved by the Food and Drug Administration (FDA) and a civilian market exists for that product, the matter is straightforward: DoD enters the market as one purchaser among many and obtains what it needs at the market price—a relatively simple transaction. Military purchase of influenza vaccine is an example. However, when the market is limited primarily to military use, even for a drug or biological that is FDA-approved, DoD's role as purchaser becomes more complicated. In the case of adenovirus vaccine for preventing upper respiratory disease among military trainees, DoD's inadequate market led the single manufacturer to cease production (Committee on a Strategy for Minimizing . . . , 2000).

DoD is not just another purchaser of drugs and biologics in a commercial market. It must also obtain drugs intended primarily for military use, such as biologics for protection against CBW agents and drugs for treating exposure to such agents. In this case, DoD assumes a second responsibility, that of a developer, as the commercial market for military use–only drugs is small or nonexistent. Under these circumstances, DoD requirements for drugs and biologics for CBW defense involve the department—directly or indirectly—in the full spectrum of research, development, clinical trials, production, acquisition, issues of medical indications of use, and postimplementation surveillance.

It was once said of the ancient world that "all roads lead to Rome." In the same way, all critical functions in the development and acquisition of drugs and biologics in the United States lead to and through FDA. The agency regulates drug development in the premarket approval stage, prescribing both preclinical and clinical research, including the protection of human subjects, in all stages, from animal studies through initial testing in humans to application for approval to market a product. FDA also regulates drug use in the postmarketing stage through required reporting of adverse events and constraints on the promotion of unapproved uses. Finally, it regulates manufacturing in both pre- and postmarket-approval stages.

At the heart of the DoD acquisition process for drugs and biologics, then, are FDA requirements that must be met before a drug or biologic may be authorized or released for human use. This reality creates for DoD a dependence on FDA, another government agency, in meeting its national security requirements for CBW defense. The management of this external dependence necessitates that DoD establish and maintain ongoing, productive relations with FDA, which involves understanding FDA regulatory requirements and incorporating this knowledge into DoD policies, organization, budgets, and procedures. Lack of such understanding can severely limit DoD's achievement of its objectives. The department's personnel involved in the acquisition of CBW drugs must be competent by education, training, and experience in their understanding of FDA policies and procedures and how they constrain or facilitate the acquisition of anti-CBW drugs and biologics. DoD must also be organized to effectively manage this dependence. It is important, then, that FDA relations receive explicit, continuing attention at both policy and operations levels.

In the course of this study, we identified three main interactions between DoD and FDA related to the acquisition of drugs and biologics for CBW defense: (1) FDA licensing of new anti-CBW drugs, (2) the use of Investigational New Drugs (INDs) in combat situations, and (3) manufacturing issues. These interactions are the focus of this report and are addressed at length in the following chapter.

A MATTER OF PERSPECTIVE

"Where you stand [on an issue] depends on where you sit" is an old truism of public administration. It is essential, therefore, to clarify at the outset the perspective we bring to this examination of DoD-FDA interactions. The literature on commercial drug development emphasizes the complexity and uncertainty of research and development, especially clinical trials, and the FDA regulatory requirements for safety and effectiveness that a new drug must meet before being approved for marketing. The preoccupation with research, product development, and FDA regulatory review is understandable, given the dominance of the pharmaceutical industry in drug development. The product development perspective is one to which the DoD is not immune.

It is important to understand, however, that FDA's view of drug and biologic development is framed by the Federal Food, Drug, and Cosmetic Act (FFDCA), which regulates therapeutic products sold in interstate commerce, and by the Public Health Service Act (PHSA), under which vaccines have long been developed. Neither the FFDCA nor the PHSA was written with the use of such products to protect U.S. military personnel against CBW threats in mind. Not surprisingly, both as a function of statute law and of actual workload, FDA is oriented primarily toward the for-profit pharmaceutical, biotech, and medical device industries. It has not been oriented strongly over time toward national or homeland security needs, although it has added personnel to deal with bioterrorism in the wake of September 11, 2001. The focus of this report is on the defense side of the DoD-FDA relationship, but we recognize that some reorientation of FDA may be needed to balance the agency's orientation toward commercial drug development and the needs of national and homeland security. We do not examine FDA understanding of DoD directly in this report. However, we believe that improving how DoD interacts with FDA, the first priority in clarifying these interactions, will result in improvements in the other direction as well.

BACKGROUND

This report concerns the acquisition of drugs and biologics for CBW defense and the related interactions between DoD and FDA. Although both drugs and biologics are included, the major concern is with vaccines, or prophylactic agents. The emphasis on vaccines stems from several factors. Historically, it grows out of the conclusion reached after the Gulf War that DoD had greater capabilities in chemical defense than in defense against anthrax, botulinum toxin, and other biological agents (Doesberg interview, 2001). In addition, vaccines provide advance protection against biological warfare threats via immunization of at-risk troops, whereas drugs are useful mainly in immediate pretreatment against certain chemical agents and in treating exposed troops. Finally, vaccine development is more complicated than drug development: Vaccines are harder to characterize than drugs and are less stable, and quality control must be applied to product, process, personnel, facility, and equipment, not just to the end product as it is for drugs.

Various external factors complicate DoD vaccine acquisition: economic incentives for vaccine development are weaker than those for pharmaceuticals; the vaccine industrial base is small and unstable; manufacturing is more difficult than for drugs; and rapidly changing vaccine science simultaneously provides the technical basis for increasingly rigorous FDA regulation and economic disincentives for the capital investment needed to respond to changing regulatory requirements. First, the market for biologicals is modest, accounting for less than 10 percent of drug industry revenues: Domestic U.S. sales in 1999 for all biologicals, including vaccines, were $6.7 billion of the $101.5 billion sales for all pharmaceuticals (Mercer Management Consulting, 1995, p. 7). Government purchases of *all* drugs and biologicals are a small part of the commercial market, accounting for less than 3 percent of all U.S. sales of human-use drugs in 1999; government purchases of vaccines are a very small portion of total drug purchases; and the military purchases of both are even smaller (Pharmaceutical Research and Manufacturers of America, 2002, Table 11, p. 127, and Table 13, p. 129). Officials at the Defense Supply Center Philadelphia, which buys FDA-licensed drugs and vaccines for DoD, estimate total DoD vaccine purchases at no more than $30 million annually (Fileccia interview, 2001; McManus interview, 2001).

Second, the vaccine industry is small and unstable. It basically consists of four major pharmaceutical firms; many smaller, older vaccine manufacturers; and a number of biotech firms. In 2001, the dominant vaccine manufacturers in the U.S. market were Merck, Aventis Pasteur, Glaxo, and Wyeth-Ayerst (now Wyeth). Annual vaccine sales for these four firms are in the $1 billion range for each of the first three companies and around $500 million for Wyeth. Recent reports, such as those on the shortage of influenza vaccine, indicate that these firms confront a number of problems in vaccine production. A number of smaller firms hold FDA licenses for vaccines based on technology from earlier eras and face disincentives, including prohibitively high capital costs, to upgrade production capabilities to current standards. The third vaccine industry segment consists of biotech firms pursuing newer approaches to vaccine development (few of which have brought licensed products to market).[2]

Third, the costs of developing new drugs and vaccines are very high. Recently the Tufts [University] Center for the Study of Drug Development estimated the cost of developing a new drug at $802 million, updating a 1987 estimate of $287 million (Tufts, 2001). Cost estimates per vaccine were estimated by a DoD expert panel in 2000 at $300–400 million for research and development, $75–115 million for capital investment, $30–35 million per year for annual operating expenses, and 5–10 percent per year for infrastructure investment (DoD, 2000, pp. 16–23). An Institute of Medicine study that polled experts on the probable research costs for 26 vaccines generated cost estimates in the range of $120–360 million per vaccine (Stratton, Durch, and Lawrence, 2000, pp. 54–55). DoD's budgets for primarily developing and licensing vaccines have not reflected these estimates. In addition, the pharmaceutical industry may not want to work with DoD, because DoD does not have easily predictable requirements; does not execute buys efficiently; is unwilling to make enough investments to maintain current Good Manufacturing Practice (cGMP) facilities; and is not a reliable customer and thus may not represent a long-term relationship. Moreover, larger companies do not want to deal with inspections under the Chemical and Biological Warfare Conventions. The companies do not want to have to submit to inspections, which may disclose trade secrets and lessen industrial advantages (Armbruster interview, 2001).

DoD, then, is a minor customer in a specialized niche market of minimal commercial interest. The needs of homeland security may expand the potential for a dual-use military and civilian market, but that has yet to occur. Public-sector financing may be required, therefore, to a greater extent in the development of CBW drugs and vaccines than for general military health needs.

---

[2]The industrial base of the vaccine industry presents challenges to DoD acquisition. The absence of a vaccine production capability adequate for meeting national needs is one reason, in 2001, the Institute of Medicine called for a national vaccine authority and the Gilmore Commission recommended creation of a government-owned, contractor-operated vaccine corporation.

In the early and mid-1990s, DoD responded organizationally to the vaccine issue by creating the Joint Program Office for Biological Defense (JPO-BD) and establishing the Joint Vaccine Acquisition Program (JVAP) within that office. The perceived limitations of the JPO-JVAP organization have led some to advocate the creation of a government-owned, contractor-operated (GOCO) vaccine production facility or its equivalent. In addition, both the Gilmore Commission and the Institute of Medicine have advocated for the creation of a GOCO for vaccines (Gilmore Commission, 2001, p. 9; Council of the Institute of Medicine, 2001). In Congress, legislation is under consideration to pursue a different strategy—one that would provide economic incentives for a biodefense industry, including vaccines—that encompasses tax, liability, and intellectual property considerations.

Although there are broader policy issues related to the acquisition of drugs and biologics for CBW defense than those examined in this report, this report is limited to the important but often overlooked issue of DoD-FDA interactions. RAND undertook this study for the Office of the Deputy Assistant to the Secretary of Defense for Chemical and Biological Defense (DATSD[CBD]). Our purposes were (1) to examine the interactions between DoD and FDA as they affect the development and acquisition of drugs and biologics for CBW defense and (2) to identify potential improvements in those interactions as they affect future CBW defense needs.

Parenthetically, we note that vaccines developed mainly for military use are also effective against naturally occurring infectious diseases, not just biological warfare threats. Consequently, we consider briefly later in the report the merits of separating vaccines for biological warfare defense from those used against naturally occurring infectious diseases. Changing this artificial separation will require legislation by Congress. Because vaccines for biological warfare threats have potential use against bioterrorist attacks on the U.S. domestic civilian population, coordination of military and civilian vaccine development is also considered in this report.

ORGANIZATION OF THE REPORT

The following chapter deals with the three acquisition challenges in DoD-FDA relations: licensing, the use of INDs in combat, and manufacturing. Chapter Three examines the industrial model of drug development, emphasizing the high-control strategy over all aspects of product development, especially for vaccines; looking at the deep investment by private pharmaceutical firms in education and training (E&T), especially as related to manufacturing; and highlighting the fact that relations with FDA are managed as a high-level corporate function. In Chapter Four we make recommendations first about E&T of DoD personnel related to FDA regulation and then about organizational changes to strengthen Office of the Secretary of Defense (OSD) policy oversight of relations with FDA regarding drugs and biologics for CBW defense.

RESEARCH METHODS

The study examined the pertinent sections of the two relevant statutes, the FFDCA and PHSA, and their implementing regulations in the Code of Federal Regulations Title 21 (21 CFR). We searched the literature for relevant documents, especially for the type of pertinent reports that seldom get entered in the archival literature.

In addition, we interviewed approximately 64 individuals in DoD, FDA, the pharmaceutical industry, academia, and related organizations. A list of those interviewed can be found at the end of the report. Within FDA, we interviewed officials in the Center for Biologics Evaluation and Research (CBER), which has primary responsibility for vaccines and other biologics. We also interviewed officials in the Center for Drug Evaluation and Research (CDER), the larger of the two centers, which has responsibilities for pharmaceutical drugs. In the private sector, we interviewed individuals in both the pharmaceutical development industries and in the for-profit and not-for-profit pharmaceutical E&T establishment.

Our initial expectations were that we would interview far more FDA officials than we did. However, we ended up interviewing more DoD officials, at all levels of policy and operations. Officials were interviewed in the following DoD offices: Anthrax Vaccine Immunization Program (AVIP); J-4 Logistics Directorate; Office of the ASD(HA); JPO-BD; the Defense Supply Center in Philadelphia; Office of the Assistant to the Secretary of Defense for Nuclear, Chemical, and Biological Defense Programs; U.S. Army Soldier Biological and Chemical Command; U.S. Army Medical Materiel Development Activity; and U.S. Army Medical Research Institute of Infectious Diseases

(USAMRIID). This wide range of interviews occurred for several reasons. First, we encountered a very complex, decentralized, and fragmented organizational system for drug and vaccine development. This required us to understand the relation of different DoD organizations to CBW drug and biologics development and the relation of these organizations to FDA. Second, few of those we interviewed had a comprehensive view of DoD-FDA relationships, and this reinforced the need to interview broadly. Third, unlike certain policy research issues, such as military manpower, that have been studied continuously for several decades by researchers with established clients, the issue of DoD-FDA relations does not have a deep history of analysis. Consequently, we faced the need to frame the issue, a task that led us to go beyond the data obtained from the interviews. Had the issue been well studied, we probably would have conducted fewer, more-focused interviews. Finally, we encountered an order of complexity in the fact that DoD-FDA relations are only one facet, albeit an important one, of a much larger problem. That larger issue is how DoD is to obtain drugs and biologics for CBW defense in sufficient quantity, in a timely manner, and at an acceptable price. Maintaining focus on DoD-FDA relations in light of broader issues of organization and finance remained a constant challenge.

Chapter Two

THE CHALLENGES OF ACQUISITION

Three primary interactions between DoD and FDA are essential to the acquisition of drugs and biologicals for CBW defense: licensing drugs and biologics for military uses, especially CBW defense; using drugs and biologics classified by FDA as INDs in certain combat situations; and ensuring that quality control of manufacturing complies with FDA's cGMP requirements.[1]

FDA regulates three types of human use diagnostic and therapeutic products—pharmaceuticals, biologicals, and medical devices—each somewhat differently.[2] It regulates drugs through CDER; biologics

---

[1]INDs are also required for laboratory personnel in, for example, the Special Immunization Program.

[2]*Drugs* are defined under the FFDCA as

> (A) Articles recognized in the official United States Pharmacopoeia, official Homeopathic Pharmacopoeia of the United States, or official National Formulary, or any supplement to any of them; and (B) articles intended for use in the diagnosis, cure, mitigation, treatment, or prevention of disease in man or other animals; and (C) articles (other than food) intended to affect the structure or any function of man or other animals; and (D) articles intended for use as a component of any articles specified in Clause (A), (B) or (C). A food or dietary supplement for which a claim, subject to sections 403(r)(1)(B) and 403(r)(3) of this title or sections 403(r) and 403(r)(5)(D) of this title, is made in accordance with the requirements of section 403(r) of this title is not a drug solely because the label or the labeling contains such a claim. A food, dietary ingredient, or dietary supplement for which a truthful and not misleading statement is made in accordance with section 403(r)(6) of this title is not a drug under clause (C) solely because the label or labeling contains such a statement.

A *biological product* is defined under the PHSA as

> A virus, therapeutic serum, toxin, antitoxin, vaccine, blood, blood component or derivative, allergenic product, or analogous product, or arsphenamine or deriva-

through CBER; and medical devices the Center for Devices and Radiological Health (CDRH). Combination products—e.g., a chemotherapeutic drug delivered to a tumor site by an infusion medical device—are evaluated by the center responsible for the dominant product in the combination. Medical devices are not considered in this report.

FDA regulation of drugs and biologics ensures that products distributed in interstate commerce are safe and effective. It represents a clear social policy designed to interrupt the flow of pharmaceutical innovation into the marketplace until evidence can be established of safety and effectiveness. Safety and effectiveness, of course, are not absolutes but reflect a judgment that the risks of a given product are outweighed by its benefits. Obtaining FDA licensure, therefore, is a major concern of pharmaceutical firms seeking to bring new drugs to the commercial market. Although such firms conduct research on not-yet-approved drugs, classified by FDA as INDs, they may not market them in interstate commerce.

DoD's interest in licensed products is that of a buyer, which differs from a pharmaceutical firm, whose interest is that of a seller. Both share a concern with moving INDs through the FDA approval process. The DoD interest stems from relative ease of use of licensed drugs and the markedly different (and substantial) recordkeeping requirements of INDs. Licensed products also avoid issues of wartime acceptance and the inevitable postwar political cost of giving military personnel products classified as "investigational" but perceived as "experimental." These factors—greater ease of use, lower recordkeeping requirements, and greater troop and public acceptance—make licensed products more attractive than INDs to DoD.

LICENSING

The regulation of drugs and biologics is extensive in scope, detailed in content, lengthy in time, and continuously evolving. FDA regulates each step of product development, including preclinical research,

---

tive of arsphenamine (or any other trivalent organic arsenic compound), applicable to the prevention, treatment, or cure of a disease or conditions of human beings.

clinical trials, labeling, testing, shipping and storage, manufacturing, postmarketing activity, and advertising of licensed products. FDA regulation is prescribed by statutes, by regulations having the force of law and by guidance documents that lack the force of law but represent the best agency thinking on a given issue.[3]

The FFDCA authorizes the regulation of pharmaceuticals. It requires that drugs not be adulterated or misbranded (1906); that sponsors provide the agency premarket notification of a drug's safety (1938); and that the agency evaluate new drugs for safety and effectiveness before approving them for marketing (1962) (Merrill, 1996). Federal regulation of biologics antedates drug regulation, as vaccines were a major public health activity at the end of the 19th century. The Biologics Control Act of 1902 authorizes their regulation under the PHSA.[4] From the end of World War II until 1970, licensing authority was held by the Division of Biologics of the National Institutes of Health. Both authority and organization were then transferred to FDA and, until recently, provided the basis for the today's CBER. Biologics are regulated under both the PHSA and the FFDCA; they are classified as drugs under FFDCA for regulatory purposes.

Preclinical testing is required before a drug or biologic may be tested in humans. This testing includes both laboratory and animal studies, which often progress from mice to primates, to generate safety data that support a request to initiate testing in humans. *Clinical trials* generate data about the safety and effectiveness of a new drug or biologic for human use and identify the patients who would benefit from the intervention. Phase 1 trials consist of the initial testing for safety, are typically short, and generally involve fewer than 20 healthy volunteers. Phase 2 trials are larger and usually involve patients with the disease or condition in question. They are undertaken to obtain preliminary information on effectiveness and additional safety data. Phase 3 trials involve study populations large enough to demonstrate benefit when compared with a placebo, are undertaken to thoroughly assess effectiveness and safety, and provide the primary data

---

[3]The CBER website on September 24, 2001, included a 12-page, 194-document list of guidance documents spanning blood, therapeutics, vaccines, gene therapy, allergenics, tissue, and devices (see www.fda.gov/cber/guidelines.htm, accessed July 2003).

[4]See, for example, Sensabaugh (1998) for a detailed examination of CBER's product review and evaluation process.

that support the product license application. All phases of clinical research require prior review by an Institutional Review Board and the informed consent of all human subjects involved.

A clinical trial of a new drug or biologic may be initiated only after the sponsor submits an IND application to FDA. The agency has 60 days in which to review whether the drug or biologic is sufficiently safe for human testing; however, a sponsor may begin testing if FDA has not responded within 30 days. The IND application provides data showing that it is reasonable to test a new drug or biologic in humans. It includes information about the composition or chemical structure of the drug or biologic; how the compound is manufactured; the methods of testing for safety (and for purity and potency in the case of vaccines); the results of prior laboratory and animal studies; how, where, and by whom the new studies will be conducted; how the drug or biologic is thought to work in the body; and any information on toxic effects found in animal studies. All the important details of the design, conduct, and proposed analysis of the clinical trial are provided in an IND and in amendments to the IND as testing progresses through successive phases of development.

Vaccine regulation is similar to drug regulation in many ways and more stringent in others. The biologic regulations are codified 21 CFR: Preclinical studies must be conducted according to Good Laboratory Practices (GLPs); clinical studies in accordance with Good Clinical Practices (GCPs); and manufacturing must comply with the current cGMPs that apply specifically to vaccines and other biologics (Ebbert, Mascolo, and Six, 1999; Parkman and Hardegree, 1999).

The data generated in Phase 1, 2, and 3 clinical trials provide the basis for a sponsor's application for a product license to market the drug or biologic. The application for a new pharmaceutical is known as a New Drug Application (NDA); that for a biologic is a Biologic License Application (BLA).[5] A multidisciplinary internal FDA team of scientists reviews the application, which must provide sufficient

---

[5]The BLA was established pursuant to the Food and Drug Administration Modernization Act of 1997, consolidating a prior requirement for two applications: a Product License Application and an Establishment License Application. The final implementing rule reduced the amount of information a manufacturer is required to file in its BLA application and shifted responsibility to the plant inspection process to ensure that manufacturers complied with cGMP standards.

information for the reviewers to evaluate safety and effectiveness and analyze whether the benefits of the product exceed its risks sufficiently to warrant approval (FDA, 2001). Review of a BLA may include a surprise preclinical inspection of the manufacturer. A review also includes consideration of an NDA or BLA application by an independent external advisory committee, which examines a summary of the application and advises the agency on whether sufficient data exist to recommend licensure (Rettig, Earley, and Merrill, 1992). For vaccines, the external entity is the Vaccines and Related Biological Products Advisory Committee, whose members include representatives of the Centers for Disease Control and Prevention and of the National Institutes of Health as well as academic researchers. FDA usually acts in accord with advisory committee recommendations but is not legally required to do so.

NDA requires manufacturers to submit product-labeling language, which describes the proper use, benefits, and risks of the product in question. FDA may also require, as a condition of approval of an NDA or BLA application, that postmarketing studies be conducted to monitor and confirm the safety and efficacy of a product as it is used more widely in clinical practice. In addition, all sponsors or manufacturers are required to monitor and report adverse effects, defined as health effects that may or may not be related to the drug in question. For vaccines, adverse events that occur after immunization must be reported to the Vaccine Adverse Event Reporting System.

Because many of the agents that terrorists or states might use do not occur in nature and might be lethal or permanently disabling, pharmaceuticals to protect and treat many chemical, biological, radiological, or nuclear agents cannot ethically be tested on humans. To address this, the FDA's "animal rule" went into effect on June 30, 2002. The rule was designed to ease the approval of pharmaceuticals for the prevention and treatment of these unconventional weapons. Under this rule, some pharmaceuticals (including biologics) may be approved on the basis of human safety data, when the mechanism of toxicity and its prevention or reduction is reasonably well understood, and on animal efficacy data, when effectiveness is demonstrated in more than one animal species, the pharmacologic pathway is similar in animals and humans, and the correct dose in humans can be determined from the data. The regulation also requires postmarketing studies.

THE DEPARTMENT OF DEFENSE'S ORGANIZATION FOR FDA INTERACTION

How is DoD organized to respond to FDA licensing requirements for CBW defense? In the DoD acquisition process, responsibility for the entire product life cycle for all weapon systems and technologies at the OSD level resides with the Under Secretary of Defense for Acquisition, Technology, and Logistics. The product life cycle is organized in three stages: science and technology base, advanced development, and procurement and sustainment.

Responsibility for CBW defense has been under the department's Chemical and Biological Defense Program. Oversight for this program is provided by an OSD steering committee, acting through the Joint Service Requirements Office for Chemical, Biological, Radiological, and Nuclear Defense (replacing the Joint Service Integration Group) and the Joint Service Materiel Group. The DATSD(CBD) provides policy and budgetary oversight for the entire life cycle for medical (drugs and vaccines) and nonmedical defenses and reports to the Secretary through the Under Secretary (DoD, 2001b).

DoD organization for CBW defense changed in 2002–2003. Previously, organization for chemical and biological defense differed, with the entire chemical warfare defense product life cycle being the responsibility of the U.S. Army Medical Research and Materiel Command (USAMRMC) and the biological warfare defense life cycle being divided between USAMRMC, responsible for the science and technology base, and JPO-BD, responsible for advanced development.

In 1992–1993, when JPO-BD was established under the Defense Acquisition Board, it had two tasks, both of which responded to the biological warfare threat identified during the Gulf War. The first was the (nonmedical) task of detection of biological warfare agents, and the second the stockpiling of (medical) vaccines for use against such threats. JPO-BD has administered the Anthrax Vaccine Production Program, which is responsible for the acquisition of anthrax vaccine, and the JVAP, which has been and remains responsible for the advanced development of other biological warfare defense vaccines.

The Joint Program Executive Office for Chemical-Biological Defense (JPEO-CBD) has now replaced JPO-BD and is responsible for advanced development of both drugs for chemical warfare defense and biologics for biological warfare defense. This includes carrying candidate drugs or biologics through program definition, risk reduction, engineering, and manufacturing development and, when they reach a certain stage, contracting with a for-profit pharmaceutical or biotech firm to manufacture the product.

Since its inception, JVAP has received candidate vaccines from science and technology organizations and other sources. It exercises its advanced development responsibility through a prime systems contractor, the DynPort Vaccine Company. DynPort manages JVAP's entire vaccine development effort, including its subcontracts with other firms for specific vaccines (Danley interview, 2001). Vaccines are currently under development for smallpox, next-generation anthrax vaccine (Baker interview, 2001), plague, Venezuelan equine encephalitis, multivalent equine encephalitis, multivalent botulinum, and ricin. DynPort is also responsible for FDA licensure, which will be sought in fiscal years 2003 to 2007 for smallpox vaccine and is anticipated for all others in fiscal years 2008 to 2017 (DoD, 2001b, p. 53).

In parallel with JVAP is a new office for medical chemical defense under the JPEO-CBD. This office resulted from the transfer of the advanced development function for chemical warfare defense from USAMRMC to the new JPEO-CBD.

Two research programs (science and technology base) remain under USAMRMC, one for medical chemical defense and the other for medical biological defense. USAMRMC exercises its responsibility for these programs through the U.S. Army Medical Research Institute of Chemical Defense for chemical warfare defense and USAMRIID for biological warfare defense (Parker interview, 2001).

Neither the current nor the prior organization provides a focal point for OSD interaction with FDA (Danley interview, 2001). For example, in the critical area of vaccine development, DynPort, as a private defense contractor, is not in a position to coordinate departmental interactions with FDA. In addition, the fact that advanced development is organizationally separate from procurement further complicates DoD relations with FDA, as organizations in both domains have an interest in such interactions.

Finally, the artificial separation of vaccine development for biological warfare defense from that for naturally occurring infectious diseases, which is required by statute, further complicates DoD interactions with FDA. Although infectious disease vaccines fall outside CBW defense and have not been part of this study, a need exists for vaccines to protect U.S. troops against endemic infectious diseases in the remote places of the world to which they may be deployed. Infectious disease vaccines may have great potential use in developing countries but have no U.S. market. Although their development is very similar to vaccines for biological warfare defense, statutory provisions assign responsibility differently for biological warfare defense vaccines than those for infectious diseases. A recent report to the Deputy Secretary of Defense argued for combining vaccine development for biological warfare defense and infectious diseases in a single entity (DoD, 2000, p. A-1).

What characterizes DoD drug and vaccine development as related to CBW defense? First, many organizations are involved, which is a source of complexity in its own right. Within OSD, the authority of the DATSD(CBD) for acquisition is limited to policy and budgetary oversight and does not include operational control over the elements for which the office must answer to the Secretary of Defense and Congress. This separation of policy oversight from operational authority contrasts with the high-control industrial model of drug and vaccine development described in Chapter Three.

Second, responsibility for the product development life cycle for biological and chemical warfare defense, although more coherent organizationally than before, still separates research from development. This complicates the handoff from laboratory to clinical studies, from clinical studies to manufacturing, application for FDA approval, and licensure. Unlike the control exercised in most commercial drug development, the various transitions in this complex process involve the transfer of responsibility across several organizations, for example, from one government laboratory to a development agency and from there to an external contractor. For biological warfare–related vaccines, for example, control of a given vaccine candidate through the product development process is transferred from an USAMRMC research project to a JVAP development project; from there it is contracted to DynPort for product development, preparation, and submission of a BLA to FDA; and DynPort may further subcontract these functions to another firm for a specific vaccine. Control over the entire process is fragmented within the government and between the government and the private contractor. The organizational pattern is shared control, not high control, even though biological warfare defense vaccines are a high priority (Danley interview, 2001).

Third, as the anthrax vaccine experience reveals, both DoD acquisition personnel and the contractors hired by DoD have not always possessed the technical and managerial expertise for working with FDA.[6] Interactions with FDA, especially in licensing-related efforts, involve a complicated three-way relationship among DoD, the private contractor, and FDA. This relationship is quite unlike either the two-way relationship between DoD and defense contractors involved in the procurement of weapon systems or the two-way interaction between FDA and a private drug firm. The policy and operational issues about how to manage these three-way relationships have yet to be worked out.

Fourth, limited resources have been allocated to CBW drug and biologic acquisition.

Finally, technical models for approval of vaccines that cannot be tested on human subjects for efficacy and must rely on animal studies are only now being developed empirically.

USING INVESTIGATIONAL NEW DRUGS

Historically, many vaccine candidates developed by DoD researchers primarily for military use, including those for CBW defense and for protection against infectious diseases, enter the initial IND stage of phase 1 studies but never progress through phase 2 and phase 3 clinical trials to the point of NDA/BLA submission. They are never licensed by FDA but simply languish in the IND state (Clawson interview, 2001). Three factors account for the infrequent licensing of these drugs and vaccines. First, the small markets for such military use products provide inadequate economic incentives to private pharmaceutical firms to drive such compounds through the entire

---

[6]Doesburg interview (2001); Balady interview (2001); Cox interview (2001).

product development and licensing process. Second, DoD is not well organized or budgeted to take drugs and vaccines through the lengthy, costly, and uncertain process. Third, unlike commercial products, human testing of the effectiveness of a drug or vaccine for CBW defense is precluded on ethical grounds because it would expose individuals to the potentially lethal chemical or biological agent in question.

On the latter point, FDA has promulgated a rule (the animal rule) that allows alternatives to human testing for effectiveness and relies on surrogate endpoints. The regulation was originally proposed on October 5, 1999, and went into effect on June 30, 2002.

The net result of these three factors is that many drugs or vaccines simply remain in IND status for indefinite periods. The IND (or "not yet approved" for human use) status may mean that the product in question is genuinely experimental. Or it may simply mean that it has not been licensed because an NDA or BLA has never been submitted. However, in some cases a not-yet-approved drug or vaccine may be the "best available" treatment—better than no treatment or better than an approved treatment of limited effectiveness—for a very specific medical use. This is true for certain drugs or vaccines for countering CBW threats, for which DoD holds the INDs. (It is also true for certain public health vaccines, in which the IND is held by the Centers for Disease Control and Prevention.)

Normal FDA licensing decisions involve a risk-benefit analysis, weighing whether the therapeutic or prophylactic benefits of a drug or vaccine exceed the risk of use. In the case of drugs and vaccines for CBW defense, the appropriate risk-benefit analysis against the prospect of the use of CBW agents by a known enemy in an active military conflict must also include the risk of nonuse. Failure to use the "best available" treatment, even if it has not yet been approved (i.e., licensed) by FDA, may leave military personnel unprotected against lethal CB agents.

However, severe constraints do exist on DoD use of IND drugs and vaccines for CBW defense in military combat. The issue of IND use arose in the Gulf War in the case of pyridostigmine bromide (PB), which was regarded as the most effective pretreatment against exposure to the nerve gas Sarin, and pentavalent botulinum toxoid (BT) vaccine, which was the most effective prophylactic against botulism. Although PB was an FDA-licensed drug for treatment of myasthenia gravis (in much higher doses and for much longer durations than those recommended for use in the Gulf War), it was classified as an IND for the indication as a nerve gas pretreatment. BT was also classified as an IND and had been used for several decades to protect certain agricultural and industrial workers.

Consequently, anticipating the need for the potential use of PB and BT in conflict with Iraq, and wishing to comply with FDA regulations, Enrique Mendez, Jr., ASD(HA), sought FDA authorization to waive the informed consent requirement for these two drugs in October 1990, on the eve of the Gulf War. He did so on the grounds that obtaining informed consent in an active military conflict was neither feasible nor desirable in protecting individual soldiers, military units, or strategic capability. FDA responded by issuing an Interim Rule in December authorizing the Commissioner of Food and Drugs to grant such waivers; under this authority, the Commissioner granted requests in early January 1991 for time-limited waivers of informed consent for both PB and BT (Rettig, 1999).

The rapid issuance of the Interim Rule by FDA in 1990 and the granting of waivers under the rule in 1991 created an expectation within DoD, which was communicated to FDA, that a final rule would be issued soon after the conflict. However, FDA delayed acting throughout the 1990s, despite the encouragement of a presidential commission. In fact, it was about to revoke the rule entirely in 1998 when the controversy was resolved. Legislation was enacted without hearings or consultation that retained the authority to waive informed consent for the use of IND-classified products in military contingencies but removed authority for such waivers from the FDA Commissioner and vested it in the President of the United States. Future waiver requests were to be submitted to the President by the Secretary of Defense, not by the ASD(HA). The President, in reaching his determination on a waiver request, was obligated to rely on rigorous regulatory criteria specified in FDA regulations and to stipulate requirements for DoD implementation of waivers in accordance with those regulations (Thurmond Act, 1998). The practical effect of this legislation has been to raise the bar for deciding to use INDs and for waiving informed consent to the level of a presidential decision, which is not inappropriate given the stakes involved. Although the country has not faced a military conflict in which the implementation of this statute has been tested, the law diminishes the willingness of the military to use anything but licensed drugs in future conflicts.

What is wrong with relying on an inventory of IND drugs and vaccines for CBW defense? There are three problems. First, the ease of use of licensed drugs is substantially greater than the ease of use of not-yet-approved drugs. The decision to use the latter must now be made by the President of the United States, the highest political authority in our constitutional system of government, whereas the decision to use licensed drugs can be made by medical personnel at the field command level. A starker contrast is difficult to imagine. A medical decision involves the expected compliance of military personnel with orders from higher authority and is grounded in the need to provide individual and collective protection in the face of enemy threats. The political decision involves a complicated process of deciding to use not-yet-approved drugs and waiving informed consent to do so, a decision vulnerable to substantial second-guessing.

Second, the use of INDs in military contingencies requires burdensome recordkeeping. Notwithstanding the authority granted by the Commissioner to waive informed consent for PB and BT, the U.S. military failed to comply with the extensive IND recordkeeping regulations: FDA review of information provided to individual recipients of IND drugs, medical monitoring and reporting of the use of such drugs, information about shipment and storage of drugs, disposition of unused IND drugs, and submission of annual and other reports. In 1993–1994, the military again failed the recordkeeping requirements for the use of tick-borne encephalitis vaccine in Bosnia, in a situation far less complicated, in military terms, than the Gulf War. Recordkeeping constitutes a major constraint on the use of INDs in military combat, one that translates into a strong disincentive to field commanders and medical personnel to use INDs.

Third, it is nearly impossible to avoid the identification of *investigational* with *experimental* and difficult to avoid its connotations of "untested" and "unsafe." A semantic solution to this conundrum does not exist. Although the President may justify the use of INDs in actual conflict on the grounds that the benefits of IND use (or the costs of nonuse) exceed the risks, such a decision runs the risk of acceptance by military personnel at the time. It also invites post-conflict political controversy about such a decision, as the Gulf War's aftermath demonstrated.

Three problems, then, accompany the use of not-yet-approved CBW defense drugs and vaccines: ease of use, recordkeeping, and troop acceptance in conflict and political controversy in the aftermath of conflict. The problems of IND use arise, however, from the weakness of the DoD development and licensing capability. Were DoD more effective in managing the drug development and licensing process, fewer candidate drugs and vaccines would be "parked" in IND status, and more would reach licensed status. Were the acquisition system more effective in ensuring the steady progression of drugs and vaccines through the licensing process, the matter of waiving informed consent would arise less frequently and would make it easier to protect military personnel.

MANUFACTURING

Manufacturing complexity is well illustrated by the recent experience with the anthrax vaccine. Following the creation of JPO-BD in the early 1990s, anthrax was identified as the primary biological warfare threat to military personnel. Weaponized anthrax, designed to propagate the most deadly inhalational form, is a primary biological warfare threat because it is relatively inexpensive and technically easier to produce than many other biological weapons. Delay in recognizing the disease almost always results in death (Brachman and Friedlander, 1999). Moreover, perpetrators can immunize themselves before using it, thereby limiting their own risk. Anthrax vaccine, then, received the highest priority within DoD vaccine acquisition for biological warfare defense. In addition, an FDA-licensed anthrax vaccine existed, and the manufacturer held an FDA establishment license for its production.[7] JPO-BD assumed—mistakenly, in retrospect—that it needed only to determine the amount of vaccine needed, provide the

[7] In addition to anthrax vaccine, the organization was a licensed producer of diphtheria and tetanus toxoids and pertusis vaccines, adsorbed; immune serum globulin (human); pertusis vaccine adsorbed; rabies vaccine adsorbed; and tetanus toxoid, adsorbed. See Plotkin and Orenstein (1999), Appendix 2, pp. 1190–1193.

necessary funds, and turn the matter over to defense procurement. JPO-BD saw its medical task as the acquisition and stockpiling of a licensed vaccine, not as one involving manufacturing or FDA licensure. It gave little thought to FDA relations, which were viewed as the responsibility of the manufacturer (Doesburg interview, 2001).

In December 1997, Secretary of Defense William Cohen announced a departmentwide anthrax immunization program for *high-risk* military personnel. Implementation began in March 1998. On May 18, 1998, the Secretary authorized the vaccination of *all* military forces (Cohen, 1998). Almost 2.5 million troop-equivalent doses of vaccine were required to implement the Secretary's decision, much more than had ever been produced by the licensed manufacturer in its entire history.[8] Prior to Desert Storm, the primary vaccine users had been veterinary, laboratory, and industrial workers at risk of infection, for whom an estimated 60,000 doses of Anthrax Vaccine Absorbed (AVA) were distributed between 1974 and 1989, an average of 4,533 doses per year (Joellenbeck et al., 2002). During Desert Storm, approximately 150,000 troops received 300,000 doses of AVA, without accurate recording of recipients or adverse reactions.

To meet the sharply increased demand resulting from Secretary Cohen's decision, DoD and the manufacturer concluded that increased production capacity was needed. It was decided to renovate the existing facility without a clear understanding of evolving FDA requirements that would be activated by this decision. DoD planned to rely on stockpiles of AVA during renovation; however, potency issues with the existing stockpile prevented DoD from using many of the doses. No one fully grasped the requirements for process validation or product quality.

DoD knew that BioPort and its predecessors had a long history of FDA citations.[9] In November 1996, FDA had inspected MBPI (predecessor to BioPort) and documented numerous significant deviations from its regulations and from the standards in the estab-

---

[8]A troop equivalent dose is the amount of vaccine required to provide one individual a six-shot series over an 18-month period.

[9]BioPort had begun as a vaccine product unit within the Michigan Department of Public Health. In 1995, it was converted to a state corporation, the Michigan Biologics Products Institute (MBPI), which was then sold to what in 1998 became BioPort.

lishment license. Based on these deviations, FDA issued a Notice of Intent to Revoke letter in March 1997. Although the letter did not require that production be stopped or the product be seized, it did state that the license to produce AVA could be revoked if corrective actions were inadequate. MBPI, in its strategic plan for compliance, agreed to provide periodic reports of progress toward compliance with FDA regulations. FDA agreed to review the data and monitor progress with follow-up inspections (Elengold interview, 2000).

Although aware of these FDA-related problems, DoD pushed forward with efforts to obtain the vaccine because of the perceived threat of anthrax. DoD reportedly assumed that 12 months would be required for renovation, with 6 additional months for obtaining FDA approval. During that time, it assumed that an estimated 5 million doses in storage could be used before the existing inventory was exhausted. Two problems arose. First, bringing the new production line on stream—with FDA approval—required much longer than anticipated. Second, the time for which most of the existing vaccine stocks had been licensed had expired, and it was necessary that these doses be tested anew to demonstrate continued utility before they could be released.

As it became clear that BioPort faced major FDA compliance problems with validating the existing AVA supply and meeting the regulatory requirements of a newly renovated production line, stockpiling receded in importance for JPO-BD, and production issues gained ascendance. BioPort halted all AVA production in January 1998 to begin renovation. Technically, the new line would require FDA approval of a supplemental BLA to the existing license. Practically speaking, it required a new application, the review of which would take 6 to 12 months under the best of circumstances. BioPort, when incorporated, had agreed with FDA to comply with prior MBPI commitments. In October 1998, an FDA reinspection found continuing improvement toward bringing the facility into compliance with agency regulations (Zoon, 1999).

However, a November 15–23, 1999, preapproval FDA inspection of BioPort's manufacturing renovations, which was more focused in scope and purpose than the 1998 surveillance inspections, resulted in BioPort receiving a FDA form 483 report with observations and possible deviations in some of the following areas: validation, failure to investigate, deviation reporting, aseptic processing, filling operations, standard operating procedures, stability testing, and environmental monitoring. FDA required that all these problems be resolved before the supplemental BLA could be approved (Elengold, 2001). FDA also requires lot release approval for all vaccines. Each lot of AVA, therefore, had to be tested for purity, potency, identity, and sterility, and BioPort was not authorized to distribute any lot until released by CBER. In March 2000, DoD issued a stop-work order on the 1998 AVA contract because of production problems. Not until December 27, 2001, did BioPort satisfy FDA requirements and resume production of approved product (FDA, 2002a).

How has DoD managed the manufacturing issues related to the acquisition of anthrax vaccine? First, JPO-BD initially staffed its office with mostly nonmedical personnel drawn mainly from weapon system acquisition (Cox interview, 2001). The medical mission was understood as stockpiling biological warfare defense vaccines, not as their acquisition or licensure. Consequently, JPO-BD had not acquired sufficient personnel with FDA experience or vaccine development knowledge. This was and continues to be due in part to a lack of interest from individuals with FDA or pharmaceutical industry experience (Armbruster interview, 2001) and may be a response to the relatively low pay (Balady interview, 2001), constant job and location changes, and a lack of willingness from those with experience to work on defense issues. Since then, JPO-BD has partially remedied these personnel deficiencies through on-the-job training and hiring professionals with relevant experience, but it has provided no formal training program for them or their superiors.

Second, DoD has managed the anthrax vaccine acquisition through a large number of organizations—JPO-BD (now the JPEO-CBD) and BioPort—as indicated above. This organization reflects a complicated and uncoordinated division of labor within DoD and among vaccine researchers, medical personnel, and acquisition personnel. It also reflects a diffusion of authority and responsibility in overall management of the biological warfare vaccine development effort.

Third, rather than having a coordinated approach to FDA, DoD sent many representatives to meetings between FDA and BioPort. OSD was been represented by the Office of the Assistant to the Secretary of Defense for Nuclear, Chemical, and Biological Warfare; the

DATSD(CBD); the ASD(HA); the Office of the General Counsel; Public Affairs; and Legislative Affairs. JPO-BD was present, as was the subordinate JVAP, the Army Surgeon General, and USAMRMC. In short, DoD representation involved 20 to 30 individuals from half a dozen separate agencies, none of which exercised overall departmental authority (Balady interview, 2001; Elengold interview, 2001a). Individuals from all the organizations could and did call FDA between meetings for information and to discuss issues. Eventually, Health Affairs was given the lead for the FDA discussions.

Typically, on matters pertaining to specific therapeutic products, FDA meets exclusively with sponsors of new drugs and license holders of existing drugs. The agency's general policies and procedures for meetings with sponsors are prescribed in statute and regulation and reflect the requirements of a government agency engaged in the regulation of the private, for-profit sector. Third parties are seldom included in FDA-sponsored meetings. The anthrax vaccine case departs from the norm: Monthly meetings between FDA, BioPort, and DoD were held for several years. Because BioPort is the manufacturer and license holder for the anthrax vaccine, these meetings are technically between it and FDA. However, as DoD is currently the exclusive customer for the vaccine and the primary source of financial support for BioPort, it is not a disinterested party in these discussions. Consequently, to circumvent policies that make no provision for third-party participation, FDA routinely asked BioPort on the occasion of these three-way meetings whether it wished to grant permission for DoD to attend (Fanelli interview, 2001). BioPort routinely did so for obvious reasons. In sum, anthrax vaccine acquisition highlighted the importance of manufacturing problems in vaccine development and the extensive, if unanticipated, FDA regulatory control exercised over the manufacturing process and the product (Elengold interview, 2000).

The general challenge in manufacturing biologics is that the rapid advances in biology over the past 20 years have greatly affected the methods of vaccine research, development, and production. Molecular biology has allowed scientists to clone and characterize the molecules that determine virulence and confer immunogenicity and has thus allowed the development of new vaccine strategies.

Advances in cell biology have led to a greater understanding of cellular and molecular interactions after infection.[10]

These scientific advances have led to improved vaccine target selection, increased ability to characterize vaccines more accurately, greater purity of vaccines, and improved safety and efficacy profiles. They have also fundamentally changed how vaccines are manufactured. Advances have led to improved measurements of safety, potency, purity (i.e., in parts per million of contaminants), and effectiveness. Improved measures have then been incorporated into manufacturing processes. New analytic methods are also leading to new standards for manufacturing vaccines, resulting in more-extensive vaccine characterization, improved quality control and assurance, and integration of the vaccine development and production processes.

The contrast between vaccine production in prior years and today is substantial. John Dingerdissen, former senior director of Viral Vaccine Manufacturing at Merck, characterized it in the following way:

> Twenty years ago, one grew a cell bank to a certain size, infected the cell bank with the virus, and after so many days took a batch of liquid and filtered it. That was the bulk product. Today, for rotavirus, we take a sophisticated cell bank, developed just for the manufacturing of human product. We grow it to a large volume, perhaps a hundredfold greater than prior times (for which we need plant capacity). We inoculate it with a virus, a sophisticated seed virus developed over one to two years of [research and development] to a certain controlled seed stage so it is absolutely safe. Then we take product. Much more of the manufacturing is done up front; it is more costly, more science is involved, but we get a better product. (Dingerdissen interview, 2001b)

FDA regulation of vaccine manufacturing has also become increasingly rigorous, especially in CBER inspections of biologics and vac-

---

[10]The Institute of Medicine cited eight major areas of increased scientific understanding over the past 15 years: the role of helper T cells in antibody and cell-mediated immunity as well as cytotoxicity, mucosal immunity, mucosal immune system organization, molecular aspects of virulence, design of recombinant protein vaccines, novel vaccine delivery systems, development of novel adjuvants, and vaccines against autoimmune diseases.

cine manufacturers, according to many of our interviewees. In 1998, CBER formally established Team Biologics for post-approval inspections "to focus resources on inspectional and compliance issues in the biologics area" (FDA, 2002b). (A brief description of Team Biologics is provided at the end of this chapter.) This action shifted inspection responsibility to the Office of Regulatory Affairs (ORA), which was responsible for drug and device inspections, and reduced but did not eliminate central CBER involvement in inspections. The objectives were to establish a comprehensive regulatory approach across all product lines; uniformity between CBER and FDA field offices for inspections, policy implementation, and interpretation of cGMPs; a highly trained professional workforce; clearly defined roles for CBER and ORA regarding inspections; a rapid process for resolving differences between CBER and ORA; an approach compatible with existing FDA structures and systems; oversight to ensure consistency of decisions and actions; and efficiency and evaluation of new methods of inspection and enforcement (FDA, 2002b).

How has Team Biologics affected DoD acquisition of vaccines? In the case of the anthrax vaccine, the first Team Biologics review authorized by CBER was of MBPI and its production capability. The review drew on a history of noncompliance at the Michigan site, increased the rigor of prior reviews, and contributed strongly to the problems MBPI/BioPort had in complying with cGMP regulations. Team Biologics has also retained responsibility for subsequent BioPort inspections. Team Biologics inspections have been central to the FDA review of anthrax vaccine production modernization. They will also be a major factor in all future DoD vaccine acquisitions of any complexity.

Team Biologics marks a major shift in FDA regulation toward greater stringency relative to biologics manufacturing. Moreover, although the initial FDA focus has been on biologics, drug manufacturing is also now being subjected to similar scrutiny. Recent press accounts have highlighted manufacturing problems involving Wyeth, Abbott Laboratories, Eli Lilly, and Schering-Plough (Hanford, 2002; Petersen and Abelson, 2002). For example:

- Wyeth, which entered a consent decree with FDA in October 2000 related to two of its manufacturing facilities, will reportedly spend $7 billion over five years to boost production capacity and improve compliance with FDA manufacturing rules (Hensley, 2000).

- FDA told Abbott Laboratories in May 2002 that the Chicago manufacturing facility still did not meet FDA standards, even after the firm had devoted more than two years and 1,500 employees "to the task of getting the diagnostic-equipment manufacturing plant up to snuff. Now Abbott must continue to keep a wide range of products off the market for an indefinite time" (Japsen, 2002).[11]

The heightened manufacturing standards in and the increasing severity of FDA regulations provide an economic disincentive to upgrade manufacturing capability. Many existing vaccines were licensed according to the historical standards in existence at the time of the initial Product License Application/Establishment License Application. Upgrading to contemporary manufacturing capabilities, however, requires substantial capital investment and submission of a new BLA. In the relatively small markets for vaccines, compared with drugs, these constraints can severely dampen private-sector investment in new technology.

THE THREE-WAY RELATIONSHIP

Both the anthrax experience and the general situation reveal the complicated three-way relationship among DoD, FDA, and manufacturers of drugs and vaccines. DoD is an early-stage developer, a contracting agency, and the principal customer for CBW drugs and vaccines. The private manufacturer is simultaneously a DoD *contractor* and engaged with FDA as a *sponsor* or license holder. FDA, as the regulatory agency, has a familiar and clear relationship to a sponsor-manufacturer. But DoD and FDA have no formal mechanisms for engaging each other in national security issues. Relations are managed, as in the anthrax vaccine case, in an ad hoc way. This relationship has yet to be rationalized in policies or procedures for either DoD or FDA, even though it is quite likely to arise in the future.

---

[11]See also Burton, Anand, and Harris (2002).

FDA regulates relations between itself and sponsors of drugs and vaccines. FDA regulations require the identification of specific individuals responsible for FDA relations within sponsoring organizations. The terms that pertain to these relations include sponsor, manufacturer, and responsible head. FDA defines *sponsor* as "the person or agency who assumes responsibility for an investigation for an investigation of a new drug, including responsibility for compliance with applicable provisions of the act [FFDCA] and regulations" (21 CFR 310.3[j]). A sponsor may be an individual, partnership, corporation, or government agency and may be a manufacturer, scientific institution, or an investigator "regularly and lawfully engaged in the investigation of new drugs." FDA biologics regulations define *manufacturer* as "any legal person or entity engaged in the manufacture of a product subject to license under the act [PHSA]" (21 CFR 600.3[t]). Biologics regulations also require the identification of the *responsible head* of an establishment:

> A person shall be designated as the responsible head who shall exercise control of the establishment in all matters relating to compliance with the provisions of this subchapter [Subchapter F—Biologics], with the authority to represent the manufacturer in all pertinent matters with the Center for Biologics Evaluation and Research, and with authority to enforce or to direct the enforcement of discipline and the performance of assigned functions by employees engaged in the manufacture of products. The responsible head shall have an understanding of the scientific principles and the techniques involved in the manufacture or products. The responsible head shall have the responsibility for the training of employees in manufacturing methods and for their being informed concerning the application of the pertinent provisions of this subchapter to their respective functions. (21 CFR 600.10[a])

These requirements make clear that organizational responsibility for compliance with FDA regulations is to be fixed in an identified person: one with authority to represent the manufacturer and to ensure compliance with regulations, who is competent in science and manufacturing, and who is responsible for training others in manufacturing methods. Translated, the regulations require a single point of contact between a private manufacturer and FDA. The regulations that govern organizational relations with FDA create difficulty for DoD in fulfilling its national security obligations in drug and biologic development. Why? Unlike a commercial pharmaceutical or biotech firm, DoD seldom has a direct legal relationship with FDA as a sponsor in the final stages of drug development, unlike the preclinical and early IND clinical studies for which it is often the sponsor. By the time a candidate drug or vaccine moves into development and manufacturing, however, DoD typically relies on other parties. While these other parties—manufacturers—typically have a single responsible head serving as the point of contact with FDA, DoD has no such single point of contact.

Although we have emphasized DoD-FDA relations in this study, the three-way relationship among DoD, manufacturers, and FDA adds a measure of complexity that is greater than the management issues a pharmaceutical firm faces. Although DoD is technically not responsible as a sponsor for meeting the FDA regulatory requirements, it must understand this three-way relationship to manage the acquisition of drugs and vaccines that require FDA approval effectively.

CBER TEAM BIOLOGICS

FDA inspects manufacturers of drugs, biologics, and medical devices in relation to the submission of an NDA or BLA application. But independent of application reviews, it also inspects manufacturers periodically for compliance with such agency regulations as cGMPs. Some manufacturers are also inspected because they have a record of being out of compliance with FDA regulations. On some occasions, periodic compliance inspections coincide with inspections for NDA or BLA new product applications.

FDA inspections for drugs and medical devices have typically been conducted by field office inspectors in the Office of Regional Operations (ORO) within ORA, Office of the Commissioner. This arrangement separates the inspection function from the work of the product-oriented centers. CDER, for example, has long relied on ORO/ORA for all pre- and postapproval inspections, with the single exception of bioresearch monitoring. A similar pattern has been true for CDRH.

Until recently, CBER was the only center doing postlicensure inspections and remains the only center engaged in preapproval inspections. CBER surveillance of licensed products was described in 1998 as "the inspection of manufacturing facilities for compliance with regulations, verification that product lots conform to preapproval standards and product consistency prior to their release into distribution, and evaluation of surveillance reports, such as adverse experience reports and blood fatality reports" (Sensabaugh, 1998, p. 1012).

The jurisdiction of Team Biologics is coterminous with that of CBER and includes in vitro diagnostics, allergens, vaccines, biotechnology products, and fractionated products. Its authority is set forth in its charter and two standard operating procedures: one for core team responsibilities and procedures and another for compliance (FDA, n.d.; Taylor and Masiello, 2001). The FDA Investigations Operations Manual is the essential reference document on which these documents elaborate (FDA, 2003b).

Technically, Team Biologics consists of two distinct entities: the core group and the cadre. The cadre—consisting of 130 inspectors exclusively concerned with blood and plasma—reports directly to ORA field offices. It was created in response to an Inspector General's audit and functions independently of the core group. The term *Team Biologics* actually refers to the core group.

Team Biologics relies on a specially trained group of inspectors who are physically located in regional FDA offices, who report administratively to an office in ORA, but who report for compliance purposes to a joint ORA-CBER compliance group. In July 2001, the core group consisted of 14 inspectors located at ORA offices across the country; maximum strength has been 17; normal turnover involves both loss to industry and retirement. Core group inspectors are selected by an application process; receive special training at headquarters to ensure consistency of inspections; and, at the GS-13 level, enjoy one civil service grade higher than journeymen inspectors in the field operations.

Core group inspectors are responsible for the entire "inventory" of licensed or registered biologics manufacturers, both domestic U.S. and foreign, which is still a relatively manageable number of firms. Inspectors conduct postlicensure inspections of each manufacturer on a biennial basis. Out-of-compliance firms face more-frequent inspections, and some inspections are conducted for special situations.

Although Team Biologics inspects only the biologics operations of firms and has nothing to do with pharmaceutical inspections, it tries to coordinate its work with drug inspections to minimize the impact on a firm.

Team Biologics inspectors report to an ORA Washington, D.C., office for administrative purposes only. Although this office has a central budget, which differs from most inspection efforts, it does not exercise inspection or compliance oversight. Work plans are prepared quarterly and include decisions about which firms are due for inspections.

A Team Biologics inspection normally consists of two people from the core group, who may be joined by a product specialist from CBER. Team Biologics inspectors routinely notify district offices of forthcoming inspections. They may include district office personnel in an inspection as a courtesy but do not solicit additional participation. Inspections take an average of 10 working days.

The Team Biologics report is known as an Establishment Inspection Report, which consists of a list of observations recorded on a Form 483. In the Findings section, both products and processes are discussed and various processes are rated. Inspections of both products and the establishment focus on systematic evaluation of quality. Inspection Reports may recommend warning letters, notice of intent to revoke licenses, or civil or criminal legal action.

Normal FDA inspection reports flow from a field office investigation unit to the district office compliance unit. Team Biologics inspection reports, however, are submitted to a central compliance group, a shared function of the ORA Office of Enforcement and CBER's Office of Compliance; they are not submitted to the district office. The compliance review group receiving these reports typically includes one compliance officer from ORA and one from CBER; it usually decides on regulatory action by consensus. If consensus is not obtained, the report goes to the next higher level—to the director of the ORA Office of Enforcement, the director of the CBER Office of Compliance, and the Director of Team Biologics—for decision.

Chapter Three

THE INDUSTRIAL MODEL

The challenges DoD faces in the acquisition of drugs and biologics for CBW defense can be understood better in light of industry management of FDA relations. Three aspects of industry behavior and organization bear upon DoD-FDA relations: a general principle of high control, deep investment in E&T, and management of FDA relations as a corporate function. To anticipate the conclusion to this chapter, the success of DoD in obtaining licensed drugs and biologics for CBW defense is predicated on following the industrial model, which has successfully produced hundreds of drugs and vaccines. From 1990 to 2002, FDA approved 981 NDAs, none of which were from DoD.

THE HIGH-CONTROL INDUSTRIAL MODEL

A general orientation toward high control of internal processes and external relations characterizes the pharmaceutical industry, especially with respect to vaccines. Although drug development involves a certain amount of outsourcing of both preclinical and clinical research, industry leaders in vaccine development engage in little outsourcing and exercise high control over the entire product development process. This includes treating *regulatory affairs* (i.e., the management of relations with FDA) as a corporate function.

The major reason for the high-control orientation is that manufacturing vaccines is more complicated than producing pharmaceuticals. Pharmaceuticals are chemical entities that can be described or characterized with some analytical precision; product specifications can be developed based upon such characterization; and quality standards can be applied primarily to the end product. By contrast, vaccines, which are derived mainly from whole biological organisms, are less easily characterized. Quality control and assurance must be applied to every step of the vaccine manufacturing process and to the equipment, the facility, the people, and the product. A senior director for vaccine manufacturing at Merck put it this way:

> Drugs are chemical entities, precisely measurable and controllable within close tolerances. Tolerances can be established on the product, and within these tolerances one can live with the drug. If the drug is out of specification, it is beyond these tolerable limits. It is very different for biologics. The [Code of Federal Regulations] definition is that a biologic involves the product, the manufacturing activity, the product facility, and the people. Inherent natural variability exists at every stage of the process, at every element of the system. Some variability is controllable; some is never controllable. The variability is multiple and wide-ranging. When you add [the variability] up, a drug [or] chemical person would say you have no controls. (Dingerdissen interview, 2001a)

The industrial model of vaccine development is best described in a report requested by Congress and the Deputy Secretary of Defense.[1] The study, which was asked to report "on the acquisition of biological warfare defenses," drew heavily on the views of the expert panel that conducted it.[2] The report argued that (1) threats of biological warfare and endemic infectious disease are high consequence; (2) vaccines are the lowest-risk, most-effective response to these threats;

---

[1]DoD (2000), p. ii. The Floyd D. Spence National Defense Authorization Act for Fiscal Year 2001 (Public Law 106-398), October 30, 2000, in Section 218, directed the Secretary of Defense to report to Congress by February 1, 2001, on "the acquisition of biological warfare defense vaccines" for DoD. This report was to consider the implications of reliance on the commercial sector to meet DoD requirements; the design of a "government-owned, contractor-operated" biological warfare defense vaccine development capability; a preliminary cost estimate of such a facility; a judgment, developed in consultation with the Surgeon General of the Public Health Service, of the utility such a facility would have for supporting vaccine production for the civilian sector; the effects such support would have on the needs of the Armed Forces, accompanied by an annual operating cost estimate; and the effects that international vaccine requirements might have on military needs for vaccines.

[2]Committee members included Franklin Top, MedImmune Inc.; John J. Dingerdissen, Merck; William H. Habig, Centocor Inc.; Gerald V. Quinnan, Uniformed Services University of the Health Sciences; and Rita L. Wells, Committee for Purchase from People Who Are Blind or Severely Disabled.

(3) the current DoD vaccine acquisition program will fail; and (4) a new approach is needed and feasible. The report's underlying assumptions were that the development and acquisition of vaccines, both for biological warfare defense and infectious diseases, differed markedly from drug development and acquisition and even more so from the acquisition of engineering-based weapon systems.

The judgment that "DoD's current [acquisition of vaccine production] approach is insufficient and will fail" was based on five factors (DoD, 2000, p. ii). First, the current DoD strategy contradicted the business success model: No single entity was in charge; management was diffuse; and the program was fragmented. The strategy also involved high risks: JVAP was relying on a prime systems contractor and outsourcing multiple subcontracts. By contrast, industry had brought all vaccine manufacturing in house because the risks associated with outsourcing and compliance with FDA regulations were otherwise too high.

Second, there was a lack of integration across the product life cycle. Changing patterns of industrial vaccine development required the integration of functions across the full life cycle of a vaccine "from discovery through development, manufacturing, production, procurement, storage and distribution, sustainment, and useful life" (DoD, 2000, p. 1). An integrated approach required attention to technologies, source materials, specialized equipment, product characterization, personnel quality and training, and quality control (which includes quality assurance, testing, validation, product release, licensing, and environmental monitoring).

Third, the DoD vaccine acquisition strategy lacked essential scientific oversight and talent; compensation was inadequate; and people with the required expertise were scarce. The report estimated that the effort would require 2,500 personnel of exceptional and specialized talent for each product.

Fourth, current DoD strategy captured an insufficient share of the vaccine industrial base because it lacked indemnification and long-term contracts. Weak economic incentives did not attract private pharmaceutical firms to develop military-use vaccines.

Finally, the goals and financial resources did not match, and the timetables were too short. The committee estimated resource requirements for each vaccine under development as follows: $300–400 million of research and development per vaccine (or $3.2 billion for an eight-vaccine effort), a capital investment of $75–115 million per vaccine (or more than $370 million for the first four vaccines), a 5–10 percent infrastructure investment per year, and an annual operation and maintenance budget of $30–35 million per year per product. The committee thus sought to introduce a greater measure of budgetary realism into the DoD's view of vaccine development resource costs.

The *Report to the Deputy Secretary of Defense by the Independent Panel of Experts, Vol. I*[3] proposed the following elements as "needed and feasible" in a DoD vaccine development and acquisition strategy (DoD, 2000, p. ii):

- **Personnel:** the appointment of a Vaccine Acquisition Executive (VAE), responsible for all biological warfare and infectious disease vaccines, who would report directly to the Under Secretary for Defense for Acquisition, Technology, and Logistics; a Program Executive Officer (PEO) reporting to the VAE; the recruitment of VAEs and PEOs from the ranks of scientifically and managerially talented individuals; and program managers who would report to the PEO—one for each vaccine—none of whom would have other responsibilities
- **Advisory mechanisms:** the creation of a strategic advisory board to advise the VAE and of a Vaccine Acquisition Review Council and a Defense Medical Requirements Council to advise the PEO, and a meeting between responsible DoD officials and the CEOs or COOs of major vaccine manufacturers to explain DoD's needs and to better understand the pharmaceutical industry's view of vaccine development
- **Priority, organization, and program:** the elevation of all vaccine development activity (including both biological warfare defense and infectious diseases) to Acquisition Category I priority; the use of a combination of industry incentives, prime systems contractor, and GOCO to achieve the production of several vaccines; and the establishment of an 8-vaccine program, scaled down

[3]Also known as the Top report.

from the current DoD plan for 15 vaccines, with a phased approach beginning with the initial two vaccines.

The key industrial model concepts recommended in the report were:

1. adopt industry best practices that integrate policy, product life cycle, resources, and management
2. provide adequate resources to ensure funding stability, multiyear commitments, flexible reprogramming, and a product—not a budget—orientation
3. integrate the product life cycle, including research, development, production, licensure, and sustainment
4. support manufacturing requirements of a validated process, scientific art, and team skills
5. establish accountability through a multidisciplinary management team that is collocated with discovery and development teams.

The following statement summarized the industrial view of vaccine development:

> The research, development, and acquisition (RDA) process for vaccines is extraordinarily complex, highly technical and regulated, and difficult to articulate to those outside the vaccine business in a manner that enables them to grasp the complexity, interrelationship and dependencies of the steps in the process, let alone the overall problems encountered in getting a potential vaccine from discovery to market. . . . In the absence of such understanding, it is difficult to fully assess the magnitude of the impact of regulatory requirements and scientific problems encountered during the process on a program. (DoD, 2000, p. 9)

EDUCATION AND TRAINING

Major pharmaceutical firms also devote substantial resources to train their professional workforce for dealing with FDA and complying with FDA regulations. We provide two examples: Wyeth-Ayerst and Merck. Wyeth-Ayerst Global Pharmaceuticals, North America and Puerto Rico, requires that all personnel who "participate in the manufacture and testing and distribution of drug products for human or animal administration" be "adequately trained" in cGMP (Wyeth, 2001).

The program applies to all full- and part-time regular employees, temporary employees, transferred employees, students and interns, and contractors and consultants who are performing a Wyeth-Ayerst job involving cGMP for the first time. This includes all personnel from senior directors on down (operators, supervisors, managers, plant managers, etc.) at the plant and corporate office levels who are located at all manufacturing sites in North America. The content of cGMP training includes "support of the manufacture, processing, packing, holding, testing, and distribution of drug products, including preparation, review, and approval of documents which are subject to FDA inspection" (Wyeth, 2001, p. 2).

Training is annual, follows a prescribed curriculum, involves knowledge and skills training, is thoroughly documented, and is differentiated according to type of employee. New employee orientation covers introductory cGMP; occupational health and safety; security; contamination control (for facilities manufacturing penicillin and nonpenicillin products, cephalosporins, or toxic or high-potent materials); documentation; and controlled substances, if applicable. Training evaluation is required of new and current employees. Failure of training bars employees from performing work in the given area "until adequately trained/retrained" (Wyeth, 2001, p. 7) An employee's training experience is entered into a training history. Performance criteria are rigorous (Wyeth, 2001, p. 11).

The Merck Manufacturing Division training focuses on FDA's GMP regulations (Dingerdissen interviews, 2001a; 2001b). The company has given courses for the past three years, at the direct request of FDA, for personnel at three levels. At the *operator* level—those who touch product—monthly GMP training is required. Twelve modules of one to two hours each, continuously upgraded, must be taken each year. Process-specific training, designed to link GMP with on-the-job experience, includes introduction to GMP, detailed paperwork instruction, hands-on training, and measurement or evaluation (by testing). Training in business, financial, and personnel and human relations has now been added. Educational requirements for drug manufacturing operators have not included a college degree.

Vaccine manufacturing operators have been required to have an undergraduate degree until recently, but manpower shortages are forcing change. *Supervisors and area heads,* the next level up, receive annual GMP training. Many of these individuals have grown up in the system or have prior GMP experience. They become the GMP trainers for the operators.

At the highest level, *managers and directors* must meet an annual requirement for GMP training: one day of training in GMP-related material. This level includes directors, senior directors, vice presidents, and the president of the Merck Manufacturing Division. Training material often deals with high-level case studies. Merck brings in lawyers, executives, and consultants who have helped pharmaceutical companies get back in business after experiencing difficulties with FDA. Merck E&T related to manufacturing runs all the way from the factory floor up to the president of the manufacturing division.

REGULATORY AFFAIRS: A CORPORATE FUNCTION

DoD has adopted FDA licensure as the regulatory standard to be met regardless of the organizational approach to vaccine development (DoD, 2000, p. ii). The Top report did not go much beyond proposing a "generic industry organizational model" for managing compliance with FDA. Typically, this would include a vice president for regulatory affairs. The report draws attention to the importance of dealing effectively with FDA in a single paragraph:

> The FDA has changed a great deal over the last 10 years. Personnel from the FDA's Center for Biologics Evaluation and Research (CBER) used to conducted pre- and postlicensure inspections. Due to concerns with the regulatory oversight process, the FDA recently established Team Biologics, principally consisting of field inspectors, which now conducts biennial compliance (postlicensure) inspections. In the process of change, it is commonly perceived that the focus shifted from identifying problems and finding solutions for their resolution to one of establishing absolute compliance backed up by detailed record keeping. A warning letter that is issued by the FDA to a facility today is taken very seriously by the industry. In fact, some individuals view receipt of a warning letter as the potential end of their career. *The vaccine industry considers the reg-*

> *ulatory environment to be extremely demanding but a necessary part of business and a part of their established best business practices.* (DoD, 2000, p. 9 [emphasis in original])

A better appreciation of the importance attached by the pharmaceutical industry to regulatory compliance with FDA is gained from other sources. Regulatory affairs (RA) is an important corporate function in the pharmaceutical industry that receives high-level recognition and involves several different activities. RA exercises point of control for a drug firm in all its dealings with FDA, including correspondence, meetings, and filings and submissions. RA serves a dual repository function, for all correspondence and for corporate memory and knowledge about FDA expectations. If a meeting is necessary, RA will contact FDA to ensure that the appropriate individuals in the firm meet with the appropriate FDA officials; the RA professional will attend the meeting. Similarly, on telephone calls between the firm and FDA, arrangements will go through the RA professional, who will also be a party to the conversation. As a result of being a party to all interactions with FDA, the RA professional becomes involved in strategy discussions within the firm about how best to respond to FDA. The RA function is usually organized on a product-specific basis, either by an individual IND or BLA or grouped by a medical specialty or therapeutic area. A recent indication of increasing importance of RA professionals is their quest for certification.

In addition to the RA function, there is a *quality assurance (QA) department*, which is typically the largest regulatory compliance entity. Among its functions are quality control; technical services; quality assurance; and audit. Quality control conducts testing and provides protocol documents for product release, which is authorized by the company; FDA authorizes lot release. Technical services sets up quality control tests, establishes protocols for such tests, and examines physical equipment. QA develops, examines, and signs off on batch records; develops standard operating procedures; investigates all process deviations from standard operating procedures; and develops records and corrective actions. It reports directly to the chief executive officer and chief operating officer, not through manufacturing. Facility compliance with cGMPs is a QA responsibility involving equipment calibration, recording equipment operation and maintenance, and performing environmental monitoring for sterility. Training staff in GLP and GMP is also a QA function. The independent internal audit group simulates FDA within the company. It conducts practice GLP investigations, writes up deficiencies, follows up for compliance, and audits manufacturing processes, clinical studies, and pharmacovigilance procedures. The audit group performs final product quality control, maintains the inventory of released products, and periodically tests stability. The pharmacovigilance department is responsible for collecting information about adverse drug reactions, determining whether they are serious or unanticipated (not identified in the labeling) and reporting those that are to FDA within 15 days. If they are not serious or are expected, periodic reports, typically annual, are filed.

The scale of the RA function can be understood by reference to a major pharmaceutical firm (Burlington interview, 2000). Wyeth-Ayerst Research has more than 40,000 employees worldwide, about half of whom are in the United States. Of the U.S. employees, approximately 75 percent are involved in the supply chain (manufacturing, sales) and about 25 percent are in research and development. The RA function, which is housed in research and development, consists of about 240 people organized in five groups: publications and archiving, development (related to product use or indication), chemistry and manufacturing, labeling, and advertising and promotion. QA employs about 3,000 people: About 1,500 are in quality control; 150 in technical services; 1,000 in quality assurance; and 50 in audit. Pharmacovigilance includes roughly 220 people.

Merck and Centocor (of Johnson & Johnson) organize themselves somewhat differently than Wyeth does, but representatives of each emphasize that the same functions are performed. Centocor emphasized the philosophy of relations with FDA:

> In dealing with FDA, the recognition is essential that extensive consultation is required. This begins for us even before an IND is filed. We work extensively with CBER, especially with the monoclonal antibodies branch. It is essential to have dialogue, often painful dialogue, on a continuing basis. This is based on long, scientific, and collegial discussions, as collegial as possible. The effort must build mutual trust. We deal with them on primary objectives, endpoints, methods; we tell them what has gone wrong very early. Without this kind of relationship, trouble will occur. (McCloskey interview, 2000)

Merck echoed the same view about the importance of mutual trust and collegial relations in dealing with FDA. As one official put it:

> Our philosophy is one of mutual collegial relations and respect. It is a function of the people at Merck and their ability to interact with people at FDA. We give them feedback and let them know when they have done a good job and when we have problems with them. In turn, they let us know whether our work is solid or not. (Ukwu interview, 2000)

Another official at Merck described the dynamic in this way:

> Relations with FDA are very good. We [Merck] have excellent relations. They [FDA] have worked well with us. We work very had to make relations amicable. But they sometimes become adversarial. They push. We push back. We agree to FDA requests if they are necessary to get a product approved. They sometimes use us to set a standard for others. Sometimes it works the other way. (Dingerdissen interview, 2001b)

Relations with FDA, then, are interactive for commercial firms. As vaccine science changes, and as the ability to characterize vaccines increases, manufacturing changes in response. As FDA demands higher and higher standards of quality control over product and process, industry involvement in active management of relations with the agency is monitored closely and addressed systematically. In all interactions with FDA, high control is exercised.

Chapter Four

SUMMARY AND RECOMMENDATIONS

Congress, in the National Defense Authorization Act of 2000, requested that the Secretary of Defense report on a design for a GOCO facility to produce needed vaccines (DoD, 2001a, pp. i, 1–10, A-1). This request spoke to the key issue for DoD since the Gulf War: "securing a ready and reliable access to safe and effective vaccines for use against biological warfare agents." Our report broadens the scope to include drugs as well as vaccines for CBW defense. But reliable supply is the central issue. As we noted in Chapter One, DoD's objective in the acquisition of drugs and biologics for CBW defense, or for any other use, is to obtain the desired supply of a given product at an acceptable price."

The Top committee, convened by DoD in response to Congress, focused on one major issue: organization. The committee concluded that "the size and scope of the DoD [vaccine] program is too large for either DoD or industry alone" (DoD, 2000, p. ii). It recommended an integrated approach by DoD and industry, a "generic industry organizational model," one aligned more closely with industry best practices than current organization. Although it supported the GOCO concept, the committee argued strongly for a more elaborate public-private approach to vaccine development. Others have endorsed the GOCO approach. In 2001, the Gilmore Commission[1] on homeland security recommended the establishment of a GOCO for vaccine development (Gilmore Commission, 2001, p. 9). In that same year,

[1]Officially the Advisory Panel to Assess Domestic Response Capabilities for Terrorism Involving Weapons of Mass Destruction.

the Council of the Institute of Medicine called for the creation of a National Vaccine Authority (Council of the Institute of Medicine, 2001). The organizational issue, however, is far from settled. Although DoD found support in the Top report for the GOCO concept, it also noted pointedly that "many of the Panel's recommendations are at variance with Departmental policy, the existing vaccine acquisition strategy, as well as acquisition and procurement practices" (DoD, 2001a, p. 3).

Other issues beyond organization affect the available supply of vaccines. These include the industrial base of the vaccine industry and the economic incentives required to ensure an adequate supply. The number of major vaccine producers is few; vaccines make up a smaller portion of producers' revenues than drugs do; and the strength of the industry is a matter of some concern. Crucial economic incentives include the size of the market, questions of liability, intellectual property, and the costs of complying with FDA regulations.

These broader issues—organization, industrial base, economic incentives—affecting the supply of drugs and vaccines for CBW defense are beyond the scope of this report. We have focused on only one of the complex issues surrounding drugs and vaccines for CBW defense: DoD's dependence on FDA decisions for all aspects related to the acquisition of drugs and vaccines for CBW defense. In this study, we have assumed that the DoD priority for drugs and vaccines for CBW defense is and will remain high for the foreseeable future. Given that priority, DoD's dependence on FDA in fulfilling its essential national security objectives means that effective management of FDA relationship must be a high priority. This focus means DoD will have to pay closer attention to FDA regulatory requirements than it has in the past because they affect licensing, IND use, and manufacturing. The ambitious DoD program of drug and vaccine development and acquisition for CBW defense can be realized only if DoD understands FDA and its statutes, regulations, and operating requirements and then incorporates this understanding into acquisition policies and organization.

What options does DoD have in managing FDA relations? Three basic options exist: do nothing to change the current system; establish an E&T program on FDA regulation of drugs and biologics for all department acquisition personnel, to increase expertise and understanding; and introduce organizational changes to improve DoD-FDA interactions.

NO CHANGE

Because of the threat of chemical and biological weapons that U.S. military personnel face, the do-nothing option makes little sense. Our national leaders emphasize that weapons of mass destruction—nuclear, chemical, and biological—are increasingly available. For that reason, we are persuaded that defense against CBW agents is a high priority. Priority, of course, is reflected in formal policies, budgets, and organizational strategies. De facto medium or low priority is unlikely to be announced in any formal policies but will reveal itself in budgets and organization. No change must be regarded as the default position, the position from which DoD must be persuaded to move.

EDUCATION AND TRAINING

We address potential changes to E&T first, and then deal with organizational issues. E&T of DoD personnel on FDA-related regulatory issues will promote effective relations between the two agencies. The "on the job" training that occurred in the past decade related to anthrax vaccine production is inadequate for the future, given the uniqueness of that experience and the rapid turnover of personnel within DoD. DoD needs a continuing E&T effort that is comprehensive for all functions—from research and development through manufacturing and production, acquisition and purchasing, and including medical use. The E&T program should also involve DoD officials at all levels—policy and operational—regardless of whether their dealings with FDA are continuous or episodic, frequent or infrequent. It should be comparable in quality to similar programs in the pharmaceutical industry and to what DoD routinely provides in many other areas.

The need for a DoD E&T program on FDA arises from four sources: the dependence of DoD on FDA decisions, the comprehensive nature of FDA regulation, the fact that FDA regulation is continually changing, and the limited information that each organization has about the other. We addressed the first three of these above. Regarding mutual understanding, FDA understands commercial product development in drugs, biologics, and medical devices much better than it understands national security needs. DoD agencies, in turn, often lack working knowledge of the scope and complexity of FDA and its regulations. Although the military research and development community understands FDA requirements related to research, it is less conversant about manufacturing. The acquisition community, on the other hand, procures many goods and services, from complex weapon systems to health care for military dependents, but devotes relatively little attention to drugs and vaccines. When the latter involve FDA-licensed products for which a civilian market exists, this poses no great problem. But products in the IND phase or for which the military is the primary customer are more complicated, and the need for trained personnel is much greater.

Three sources of FDA E&T programs exist: the private sector, FDA, and DoD. Many private-sector organizations conduct E&T programs on FDA and its regulatory requirements on a continuing basis. Food and drug attorneys and regulatory affairs professionals are the primary customers for these educational programs. Three such organizations, chosen for illustrative purposes, are the Food and Drug Law Institute (FDLI), the Drug Information Association (DIA), and the Regulatory Affairs Professionals Society (RAPS). Each organization sponsors many educational conferences and programs annually, and each is potentially available to contract with DoD for E&T services. Each organization publishes educational material: FDLI, for example, publishes *How to Work with the FDA* and *The Regulatory Compliance Almanac: A Guide to Good Manufacturing, Clinical and Laboratory Practices*; DIA publishes the *Drug Information Journal*, a quarterly that contains many articles pertaining to FDA; and RAPS publishes *Fundamentals of Regulatory Affairs*.[2]

FDA also has substantial educational capabilities both for internal training of its own personnel and for training external parties (Sherman interview, 2001; McNeill interview, 2001). Internal programs may be done in conjunction with other government agencies and with private-sector organizations, including pharmaceutical

---

[2]We list information about each organization in the Appendix.

firms. Externally, FDA cosponsors meetings with industry, including FDLA, DIA, RAPS, and other organizations. In addition, FDA personnel provide seminars at meetings held by FDLI, DIA, and RAPS. Examples of such courses include the following (Sherman interview, 2001; McNeill interview, 2001):

- "Reviewer Training: Introduction to the Regulatory Process," which includes an orientation to CBER, INDs, clinical studies, and postmarketing surveillance
- "Inspection Workshop," which teaches inspectors the techniques of interviewing, evidence development, communication and coordination with the manufacturer, and what to do once inside a firm
- Supplemental GMP training, which explains how to examine the physical environment of a manufacturing facility
- Team Biologics meetings specific to product areas, such as vaccines.

FDA provided DoD officials customized E&T in February 2000, which was considered useful by many of those we interviewed in both DoD and FDA.[3] CBER's Office of Communication, Training and Manufacturers Assistance presented a basic course on FDA-CBER for both DoD and the Centers for Disease Control and Prevention in response to the problems associated with the anthrax vaccine. FDA officials indicated to RAND that it was both possible and desirable for FDA to provide E&T programs responsive to DoD needs. The lack of a central point of contact in DoD to discuss needed and available E&T was viewed as a limiting factor.[4]

DoD itself supports a vast array of educational programs for professional personnel, both military and civilian, across all aspects of departmental activity. Some E&T efforts focus on FDA. Under the USAMRMC, USAMRIID's Office of Product Development and Regulatory Affairs has increased its E&T efforts markedly over the past five years. In 2000, it provided at least ten FDA-related courses ranging

[3]Balady interview (2001); Sherman interview (2001); Fannelli interview (2001).

[4]Balady interview (2001); Sherman interview (2001); Fannelli interview (2001).

from "Introduction" to "GLP Regulations" to "Principles of Pharmacology." Instructors included FDA officials, academicians, regulatory professionals, and experts from within DoD. Courses are open to all DoD agencies, but most participants come from within USAMRMC, the parent organization.[5]

USAMRMC researchers and others at Fort Detrick involved in pharmaceutical research and development can also take courses at Hood College in nearby Frederick, Maryland.[6] The college graduate school, responding to demand from Army researchers, offers a masters degree in biomedical science and a concentration and certificate in regulatory compliance. In addition to courses in immunology, virology, and biochemistry, students must complete courses in GLP, product development, GCP, and GMP.

In addition to E&T efforts, DoD has the potential for integrating FDA-related material into established curricula in defense acquisition.[7] For example, the National Defense University exists to educate military and civilian DoD leaders. It includes the Industrial College of the Armed Forces (ICAF), whose mission "is to prepare selected military officers and civilians for senior leadership and staff positions . . . with special emphasis on acquisition and joint logistics." ICAF offers both an Acquisition Core Course and a Senior Acquisition Course.[8] Active-duty military and visiting senior civilians from federal government agencies augment a permanent faculty.[9] ICAF is a natural site for E&T related to FDA regulation, drug and vaccine development and acquisition, and DoD-FDA interactions. Many other entities within DoD might also be enlisted in E&T related to FDA. While these

---

[5]Pace-Templeton interview (2001). Dr. Pace-Templeton subsequently provided the authors with significant written information about coursework provided by USAMRIID and Hood College.

[6]For more information, see www.hood.edu/graduate/gbiomed.htm and www.hood.edu/graduate/gbioreq.htm#RCCert (accessed during the time of research).

[7]See www.defenselink.mil/other_info/education.html (accessed July 2003).

[8]See www.ndu.edu/icaf/mission/mission.htm (accessed July 2003).

[9]Participants in the Senior Acquisition Course take the ten-month ICAF curriculum plus two required elective courses dealing with acquisition policy issues. Services and agencies select students. Military officers are selected as part of the senior service school selection process by their Defense Acquisition Career Manager, according to www.ndu.edu/icaf/departments/acquisition/sac/sachome.htm (accessed July 2003).

sources exist, acquisition personnel report that they are not given sufficient time to attend even one FDA-related E&T course per year. Time for continuing E&T must be expanded, and attendance must be encouraged.

Establishing an effective E&T program, however, is difficult for high-level acquisition personnel. These decisionmakers are very busy; the acquisition of pharmaceuticals is not their primary mission; they have limited knowledge of and experience with FDA; and they have little time and are likely less willing to participate in a general E&T program that lacks an immediately discernible benefit. Moreover, they are unlikely to find E&T attractive in real-time crisis management. However, such personnel must deal with FDA in making procurement decisions about drugs and vaccines of unique military interest, especially when such decisions become matters of secretarial interest. We see no easy solution to this challenge.

This report takes the FDA regulatory regime as a given. It argues that DoD needs to know more about FDA to manage the development, production, and licensing of drugs and vaccines for CBW defense more effectively. However, we acknowledge that DoD needs to go well beyond this assumption and actively engage FDA in defining a national security agenda for drug and biologics development. The CBW threat, both to national and homeland security, raises the question of whether regulation developed for commercial drug development is adequate to meet new national needs (Javitt, 2002). Although the answer to this question is not obvious, the question itself urgently needs to be addressed.[10]

How might a drug development regulatory agenda be developed? DoD and FDA could organize an annual one- or two-day meeting dedicated to the general issues involving the two organizations as they pertain to CBW defense. This conference should not focus on product-specific issues because this would infringe on the immediate regulatory process. The broader issues that we have in mind include the following:

---

[10]RAND hosted a workshop December 19, 2002, titled "FDA and the Common Defense," with participation from FDA, DoD, the pharmaceutical industry, and others, to address some of these issues.

- scientific, clinical, and methodological issues associated with the limitation on clinical trials of CBW defensive agents arising from the ethical prohibition of exposing humans to potentially lethal compounds[11]
- the respective risk evaluation philosophies of DoD and FDA for dealing with CBW agents—i.e., whether there are persuasive arguments for a lesser standard of safety when dealing with a CBW threat than when dealing with disease and illness challenges of civilian personal health
- risk communication issues associated with the prospective administration of IND-status drugs and vaccines against CBW threats to protect military personnel when licensed products are not available
- protection of the integrity of the FDA review process from governmental bureaucratic politics if and when a GOCO for vaccine development is authorized and established
- recruitment and retention of high-quality personnel, both military and civilian, with drug and vaccine development knowledge, experience, and technical competence and the associated experience in dealing with FDA.

For such a meeting to be productive, DoD and FDA would need to develop the agenda jointly. Representatives of the civilian agencies of the federal government, such as the National Institutes of Health and the Centers for Disease Control and Prevention, as well as industry representatives, might also participate.

In short, we recommend that DoD establish a continuing E&T program on FDA and its regulatory authority, policies, and procedures for all personnel involved in the acquisition of drugs and biologics for CBW defense. This E&T effort should be pursued regardless of the strategic and organizational approach to CBW defense that DoD chooses.

---

[11]These might involve implementation of the animal rule, such as animal challenge studies, and surrogate endpoints for CBW defensive agents.

ORGANIZATIONAL CHANGE

Private-sector experience indicates that a strong E&T program is necessary but not sufficient for the successful development and manufacturing of FDA-approved pharmaceuticals. The critical DoD-FDA interactions identified in this report related to the procurement of drugs and biologics for CBW defense are (1) FDA licensing of CBW drugs and biologics, (2) determination of medical use of INDs for CBW defense, and (3) manufacturing. Of these, the FDA licensing function is central, since success in this will reduce dependence on IND use. The investment in research and development is essential, but the department needs to bring a sustained acquisition perspective to FDA relations. Manufacturing may also be very important, as we are reminded specifically by the anthrax vaccine case and more generally by the increasing regulatory attention given to it by FDA.

At present, no central authority exists within DoD for coordinating relations with FDA across all activities related to CBW defense. OSD is represented by both the DATSD(CBD) and the ASD(HA). JVAP has a small staff that deals with FDA relations but relies mainly on its prime system contractor, the Defense Vaccine Contractor, for managing FDA interactions. USAMRMC relies on its own personnel for FDA relations in the early stages of research and then hands this responsibility off to its contractors (i.e., pharmaceutical firms) in later stages. These arrangements raise questions about DoD oversight of contractor firms to ensure that relations with FDA are managed effectively. More fundamentally, these arrangements make apparent the fact that the line of authority from OSD to the defense agencies and officials managing FDA relations remains absent.

One option for DoD is to continue to rely on existing arrangements for managing FDA relations. This would involve continued reliance on pharmaceutical and biotech firms as defense contractors to manage clinical trials, product development, manufacturing, and FDA licensure. Such reliance is especially problematic for vaccines: Legacy manufacturers, such as BioPort, licensed in a different era and characterized by old plants, and equipment, are not well suited to provide vaccines in the modern era. Modern biotech firms have yet to establish a strong record of bringing new products through FDA licensing to market. (FDA approval in December 2002 of MedImmune's Flu-Mist vaccine for influenza is a very recent exception.)

And major the pharmaceutical firms producing vaccines have difficulties of their own. This status quo course has not resulted in any licensed CBW products in the past decade. Thus, the United States faced the prospect of a second war with Iraq in 12 years with no additional licensed drugs or biologics for responding to the threat of chemical or biological warfare agents.[12] For DoD to choose this pathway was to perpetuate the weak lines of OSD authority and risk dealing with secretarial acquisition decisions, which invariably involve FDA, being made by officials with little prior knowledge, experience, or training relevant to FDA regulations.

We make three recommendations. First, we recommend that DoD consolidate authority for all interactions with FDA related to drugs and biologics for CBW defense in a single OSD office. There are two candidates for this responsibility: the Office of the ASD(HA) and the Office of the DATSD(CBD). The Health Affairs option has the advantage of emphasizing medical indications for use, both for licensed drugs and for IND-classified drugs. This function is currently vested in this office, and Health Affairs should retain the primary OSD authority for this purpose. Physicians should be in charge of a medical function.

We do not minimize the importance of the determination of medical indications for use of not-yet-approved CBW drugs and biologics. Policy authority in this domain is appropriately assigned to Health Affairs. We reaffirm the importance of this OSD responsibility and do not support any infringement on this essential function. However, there are two reasons for not locating OSD authority for managing FDA relations in Health Affairs. The office has neither research and development responsibilities nor acquisition responsibilities. It is the latter that needs OSD attention, and vesting primary OSD authority for FDA relations in Health Affairs would ignore the central importance of acquisition. In addition, assigning the responsibility for FDA relations to Health Affairs would create an organizational conflict of interest that should be avoided. The office responsible for DoD medical determinations about safety and effectiveness of given drugs or biologics when used on military personnel should have the health

---

[12]FDA approved PB as a pretreatment against Soman nerve gas in February 2003 (FDA, 2003a).

and welfare interests of those personnel as its primary concern. It should not be asked to compromise its responsibility to military personnel by adding responsibility for acquisition of drugs and biologics.

The second option for the consolidation of OSD responsibility for relations with FDA for CBW agents is the Office of the DATSD(CBD). We recommend that departmental authority be vested in this office for managing when and how DoD interacts with FDA for all CBW drugs and vaccines. One potential disadvantage is that centralization of OSD authority for FDA relations risks creating a bottleneck at the top of the department. However, consolidation need not preclude the delegation of authority for specific drugs or biologics. Moreover, the volume of specific drugs and biologics for CBW defense is not large and could be easily managed. Rather, the rationale for the proposed consolidation is to clarify who speaks to FDA—that is, who speaks for the secretary and who answers to Congress—on issues of CBW defense. The primary advantage of this option is that an acquisition perspective will be brought to bear on CBW drugs and biologics from an OSD vantage point

FDA has indicated that it would welcome the recommended consolidation of authority. Early in the project, RAND met with CBER Deputy Director Mark Elengold and a number of CBER staff. The deputy director forcefully addressed the issue in the following way:

> We can't tell one DoD agency from another, [the Office of the Surgeon General] from [Health Affairs]. At a recent three-way BioPort meeting [BioPort, FDA, and DoD], we asked for one contact person to deal with at DoD. DoD was surprised at our request. We have no idea who we are talking to—AVIP,[13] Detrick, SAIC [a private contractor], JVAP. The bottom line is that DoD is no different from a large multinational drug company with many tentacles that reach to the FDA. No different from Roche or Merck. DoD needs to set up

[13]AVIP has three main responsibilities: to monitor the services' execution of the program and facilitate its execution (other than anthrax acquisition); to act as the focal point for information on the anthrax vaccine, the program, etc.; and to lead surveillance of adverse effects from the anthrax vaccine (according to Colonel Randy Randolph, Director of AVIP, interviewed July 12, 2001).

> a single RA office to manage all relations with FDA. All DoD contacts with FDA should go through the RA office. Then DoD can hire ex-FDA employees to run the RA office. In all the discussions of a GOCO, including pilot scale-up, there is no RA element. RA people understand FDA regulations and their importance. They are the ones who understand the spectrum of FDA regulatory activities and who is needed for what meeting. (Elengold interview, 2001a)

Second, we recommend the establishment of a Director of Regulatory Affairs in the Office of the DATSD(CBD) to implement the initial recommendation. Consolidation of RA authority is assumed but not elaborated by the Top report, which called for a Vice President for Regulatory Affairs. The official should

- establish general DoD policy for dealing with FDA, for all CBW defense drugs and vaccines
- function as the primary point of contact for all DoD relations with FDA for any specific CBW defense drug or biologic
- delegate operational responsibility for a specific CBW defense drug or vaccine to the appropriate DoD agency
- establish DoD general policy for relations with private contractors engaged by the department in the development of a CBW defense drug or biologic
- ensure the availability of E&T programs related to FDA and the participation of all appropriate personnel in such programs.

We must be clear, however, that we are not recommending a massive new bureaucracy in OSD but rather the designation of an official with point-of-contact coordination and control of relations with FDA.

Although this report has emphasized DoD-FDA relations, the discussion has invariably included DoD-contractor relations and FDA–drug firm relations. It has thus led to the complex three-way relationship among DoD, contractors and drug firms, and FDA. One of the important reasons for locating an RA function in DATSD(CBD) is to clarify DoD policy and procedures for managing this three-way relationship other than in an ad hoc manner. Furthermore, FDA deference to private firms when DoD has a major interest in the substance of the FDA–private firm discussions is a convention, not a sacrosanct requirement. Clarification of DoD views and policies on this issue ought to lead FDA to adapt to the needs of national security as they differ from those of commercial drug regulation.

Third, we recommend that Congress enact legislation to create comparable authority to that recommended for biological warfare vaccines for the acquisition of vaccines for naturally occurring infectious diseases within the Office of the Director for Defense Research and Engineering or that the RA officer in DATSD(CBD) be given this responsibility. Although statutory and budgetary constraints currently separate vaccine development for biological warfare from that for infectious diseases, the separation makes little sense in scientific, manufacturing, and licensing terms. Efficiencies and complementarities can be realized from treating all vaccine development for military purposes in a similar way, as the Top report argued.

CONCLUSION

The nation's senior leadership has emphasized the threat of chemical and biological weapons to U.S. military and civilians. Since the 1990–1991 Gulf War, DoD has made little progress in getting pharmaceuticals from the development stage through FDA approval, yet the threat remains or has increased. To defend our troops, changes are required, and the above recommendations reflect the authors' best judgment on changes that will enable DoD to improve its understanding of and relationship with FDA so that the approval of pharmaceuticals will be more likely.

Appendix

PRIVATE PROVIDERS OF FDA-RELATED EDUCATION AND TRAINING

The **Food and Drug Law Institute** (FDLI) is a nonprofit educational organization that publishes educational materials and sponsors conferences and workshops about the laws, regulations, and policies affecting the industries regulated by FDA (pharmaceuticals, biologics, medical devices, foods, dietary supplements, cosmetics, and animal health products). Members include manufacturers of regulated products; law firms and consulting firms involved in food and drug regulation; and associations and other service and supplier organizations. FDLI sponsors more than 20 conferences each year, most of which are one to two days long. Some illustrative conferences held in 2001 and 2002 include the following:[1]

- Introduction to Drug Law and Regulation: Understanding How FDA Regulates the Drug Industry. This conference covered the basic laws and regulations of the drug industry and provides a broad overview of FDA; the history of drug regulation, including the Food and Drug Administration Modernization Act of 1997; and specific areas of drug regulation.
- Office of Inspector General's Compliance Model for the Pharmaceutical Industry.
- 45th Annual Educational Conference, with FDA. This conference covered issues related to drugs, biologics, medical devices, and food.

[1] FDLI website (www.fdli.org), accessed November 8, 2001, and December 6, 2001.

- Academic Clinical Research: How Best to Ensure Safety and Integrity; A Legal Perspective.

The **Drug Information Association (DIA)** is a nonprofit association with more than 22,000 members from regulatory agencies; academia; contract research and contract service organizations; pharmaceutical, biotech, and medical device companies; and other health care organizations. It offers about 90 meetings and workshops worldwide each year, the majority in the United States but many also in Europe. The annual DIA meeting draws more than 5,000 participants. Some illustrative courses held in 2001–2002 include the following:[2]

- Introduction to Key FDA Meetings: Why, What, When, Where and How
- Biological Product Deviation Reporting for Licensed Manufacturers of Biological Products
- Overview of the Pharmaceutical Industry: An FDA-Industry Dialog on the Drug Development Process
- Regulatory Affairs Training Course: Part I—The IND Phase; Part II—The NDA Phase
- Global Chemistry, Manufacturing and Controls Challenges: From Drug Substance to Finished Product
- Good Clinical Practices, Audits and Surviving an FDA Inspection
- Effective Agency/Industry Interactions to Expedite Drug Development.

The **Regulatory Affairs Professionals Society (RAPS)** is a nonprofit organization providing education, professional certification, and information services to nearly 8,000 regulatory affairs professionals in government, industry, academia, and nonprofit organizations. RAPS holds approximately 30 meetings yearly. The annual RAPS conference covers a wide range of issues related to drugs, biologics, and medical devices, including privacy, harmonization, the effect of

---

[2]DIA members receive electronic and print announcements of these events. The DIA website (www.diahome.org) also posts extensive information about workshops and conferences.

research errors on clinical trials in the United States, biologic product development, and how to develop a biologics license application. Some illustrative 2001–2002 conferences include the following:[3]

- Principles and Practices of US Regulatory Affairs
- RA/QA 101: A Regulatory & Compliance Workshop
- IND Training Workshop
- FDA Inspections
- Clinical Trials: Life Cycle of a Clinical Study
- Regulatory Affairs 101.

---

[3]RAPS website (www.raps.org), accessed August 17, 2001, and November 23, 2001.

INTERVIEWS

Altopiedi, Donna, Senior Director, Global Training and Continuous Improvement, Wyeth-Ayerst Global Pharmaceuticals, telephone interview, August 9, 2001.

Arcarese, Joseph S., Executive Vice President, FDLI, February 16, 2001.

Armbruster, Vicky R., Joint Program Manager, JPO-BD, March 27, 2001.

Baker, Phillip J., Ph.D., Program Officer, Division of Microbiology and Infectious Diseases, National Institute of Allergy and Infectious Disease, National Institutes of Health, telephone interview, August 6, 2001.

Balady, Michael A., Ph.D., M.P.H., Medical Project Manager, JPO-BD, May 5, 2001.

Blanck, Ronald R., D.O., President, Health Sciences Center, University of North Texas, former Surgeon General, U.S. Army, telephone interview, October 18, 2001.

Burlington, Bruce, M.D., Senior Vice President for Regulatory Compliance, Wyeth-Ayerst, telephone interview, July 28, 2000.

Burman, Mary C., M.N., Joint Vaccine Acquisition Program, Project Management Office: Regulatory Affairs, Quality Assurance, June 27, 2001.

Casciotti, John, LL.B., Office of the General Counsel, Office of the Secretary of Defense, June 1, 2001.

Clawson, Ronald E., Ph.D., Project Manager, Pharmaceutical Systems, U.S. Army Medical Materiel Development Activity, April 19, 2001.

Clayson, Edward T., Lieutenant Colonel, U.S. Army, Program Director, Anthrax Vaccine Adsorbed Production Program, JPO-BD, telephone interview, August 22, 2001.

Clinton, Jarrett, M.D., Rear Admiral, U.S. Public Health Service, Acting ASD(HA), Office of the Secretary of Defense, April 5, 2001.

Cox, Frank, Battelle Memorial Laboratories, former Colonel, U.S. Army, Assistant to the Deputy for Chemical Warfare, Office of the Assistant to the Secretary of Defense for Atomic Energy, telephone interview, October 17, 2001.

Danley, David L., Ph.D., Colonel, U.S. Army, Project Manager, JVAP, May 1, 2001.

Dingerdissen, John J., Senior Director, Viral Vaccine Manufacturing, Merck Manufacturing Division, Merck & Co., May 31, 2001a, and July 23, 2001b.

Doesburg, John C., General, U.S. Army Soldier Biological and Chemical Command, former Program Manager, JPO-BD, telephone interview, October 15, 2001.

Douglas, Gordon, M.D., former President, Merck Vaccine Division, Merck Co., Inc., telephone interview, June 5, 2001.

Elengold, Mark A., Deputy Director, Operations, CBER, June 26, 2000; February 21, 2001a; and August 23, 2001b.

Fanelli, Winifrede L., Deputy Joint Program Manager for Biological Defense, JPO-BD, March 27, 2001.

Fileccia, Thomas C., Chief, Branch A, Pharmaceutical Business Unit, Defense Supply Center Philadelphia, July 24, 2001.

Fitzpatrick, G. Michael, Colonel, U.S. Army Medical Service Corps, Director, Armed Services Blood Program, April 5, 2001.

Friedlander, Arthur M., M.D., Colonel, U.S. Army, USAMRIID, telephone interview, August 6, 2001.

Grabenstein, John, R.Ph., Ph.D., Lieutenant Colonel, U.S. Army, Deputy Director, AVIP, July 12, 2001.

Hoke, Charles H., Jr., M.D., Colonel, U.S. Army, Medical Corps, Director, Military Infectious Diseases Research Program, USAMRMC, August 21, 2001.

Iacono-Connors, Lauren, Ph.D., Senior Advisor to the CBER Director, and Bioterrorism Coordinator, CBER, February 21, 2001.

Jennings, Gerald B., D.V.M., Ph.D., Colonel, U.S. Army, Military Assistant to the ASD(HA), OSDHA, April 5, 2001.

Korwek, Edward L., Partner, Hogan & Hartson, LLP, telephone interview, March 16, 2001.

Lynch, Kara, Deputy Director, Team Biologics, Office of Regional Operations, Office of Regulatory Affairs, OC, FDA, July 11, 2001.

Marano, Nina, Coordinator, Anthrax Vaccine Research Program, Centers for Disease Control and Prevention, telephone interview, July 11, 2001.

Mayo, Richard, Rear Admiral, U.S. Navy, Director, Logistics Directorate (J-4), Joint Staff, March 20, 2001.

McCloskey, Richard, M.D., Vice President for Medical Research, Centocor (Johnson & Johnson), telephone interview, July 31, 2000.

McManus, Stephen A., Deputy Director, Directorate of Medical Materiel, Defense Supply Center Philadelphia, July 24, 2001.

McNeill, Lorrie, Chief, Manufacturers Assistance and Technical Training Branch, Office of Communication, Training and Manufacturers Assistance, CBER, March 22, 2001.

Murphy, Diane, M.D., Director, Office of Drug Evaluation IV, CDER, March 28, 2001.

Pace-Templeton, Judith G., Chief, Product Development and Regulatory Affairs, USAMRIID, April 19, 2001.

Parker, John S., Major General, U.S. Army, Commanding General, USAMRMC, August 21, 2001.

Pierson, Jerry, RPh., Ph.D., Lieutenant Colonel, U.S. Army, Chief, Regulatory Affairs, Office of Regulatory Compliance and Quality, U.S. Army Medical Research and Materiel Command, April 19, 2001.

Plotkin, Stanley A., M.D., Aventis Pasteur, July 23, 2001.

Pierson, Vicki, Project Manager, JVAP, Project Management Office: Regulatory Affairs, June 27, 2001.

Poste, George, Dr., Chair, Defense Science Board Summer Study, 2000, on Defense Against Biological Weapons; CEO, Health Technology Networks, Health Technology Networks, telephone interview, June 20, 2001.

Prior, Stephen D., Ph.D., Research Director, National Security Health Policy Center, Potomac Institute, February 20, 2001a; June 15, 2001b; and August 15, 2001c.

Randolph, Randy, Colonel, U.S. Army, Director, AVIP, July 12, 2001.

Roeder, David, Associate Director for Regulatory Affairs, CDER (ODE IV), March 28, 2001.

Rostker, Bernie, RAND; former Deputy Secretary of Defense for Personnel and Readiness and Under Secretary of the Army, August 17, 2001.

Sherman, Gail, Director, Division of Manufacturers Assistance and Training, Office of Communication, Training and Manufacturers Assistance, CBER, March 22, 2001.

Soreth, Janice, M.D., Acting Director, Division of Anti-Infective Drug Products, ODE IV CDER, March 25, 2001.

Steele, David E., D.V.M., Product Manager, Project Management Office, JVAP, June 27, 2001.

Top, Franklin, M.D., Chair, DoD Vaccine Acquisition Study; Executive Vice President and Medical Director, MedImmune, telephone interview, June 14, 2001.

Ukwu, Henrietta, Vice President, Worldwide Regulatory Affairs for Vaccines/Biologics [also contributing to the interview was Laurence Hirsch, Vice President, Merck Research Laboratories Public Affairs], Merck, telephone interview, August 7, 2000.

Villforth, John C., President, FDLI, February 16, 2001.

Wardlaw, Butch, Communications Chief, AVIP, July 12, 2001.

Wertz, Michael M., Program Manager, AVIP, July 12, 2001.

Zadinsky, Julie, Colonel, U.S. Army, Deputy [to Major General John S. Parker, M.D., U.S. Army], Regulatory Compliance and Quality Assurance, USAMRMC, June 27, 2001.

Zajtchuk, Russell, M.D., Advanced Technology and International Health, Rush-Presbyterian St. Luke's Hospital; former Commanding General, USAMRMC, telephone interview, October 18, 2001.

REFERENCES

Alibek, K., *Biohazard: The Chilling True Story of the Largest Covert Biological Weapons Program in the World*, New York: Dell Publishing, 2000.

Arnon, S. S., R. Schechter, T. V. Inglesby, et al., "Botulinum Toxin as a Biological Weapon," *Journal of the American Medical Association*, No. 285, 2001, pp. 1059–1070.

Brachman, P. S., and A. M. Friedlander, "Anthrax," in S. A. Plotkin and W. A. Orenstein, eds., *Vaccines*, 3rd ed., Philadelphia: W. B. Saunders, 1999, pp. 629–637.

Burton, T. M., G. Anand, and G. Harris, "Leading the News: FDA Hits Abbott Labs, Schering," *Wall Street Journal*, May 16, 2002, p. A3.

Cohen, W., "Implementation of the Anthrax Vaccination Program for the Total Force," Office of the Secretary of Defense memorandum, May 18, 1998.

Committee on a Strategy for Minimizing the Impact of Naturally Occurring Infectious Diseases of Military Importance: Vaccine Issues in the U.S. Military, Medical Follow-Up Agency, Institute of Medicine, "Urgent Attention Needed to Restore Lapsed Adenovirus Vaccine Availability," letter report, November 6, 2000, published as Appendix A in S. M. Lemon, S. Thaul, S. Fisseha, and H. O'Maonaight, eds., *Protecting Our Forces: Improving Vaccine Acquisition and Availability in the U.S. Military*, Washington, D.C.: IOM, National Academies Press, 2002, pp. 107–113.

Council of the Institute of Medicine, "Statement on Vaccine Development," November 5, 2001.

Dennis, D. T., T. V. Inglesby, D. A. Henderson, et al., "Tularemia as a Biological Weapon," *Journal of the American Medical Association*, No. 285, 2001, pp. 2763–2773.

DoD—*see* U.S. Department of Defense.

Ebbert, G. B., E. D. Mascolo, and H. R. Six, "Overview of Vaccine Manufacturing and Quality Assurance," in S. A. Plotkin and W. A. Orenstein, eds., *Vaccines*, 3rd ed., Philadelphia: W. B. Saunders, 1999, pp. 40–46.

Elengold, M., Deputy Director, Operations, CBER, statement before the Committee on Government Reform, U.S. House of Representatives, October 3, 2000, at www.fda.gov/ola/2000/anthraxvaccine 4.html (accessed July 2003).

FDA—*see* U.S. Food and Drug Administration.

Fialka, J., M. Chase, N. King, and R. Winslow, "Officials Fear U.S. Is Ill-Equipped to Deal with Biological or Chemical Terrorism," *Wall Street Journal* (electronic edition), September 18, 2001, at http://interactive.wsj.com/.

Gilmore Commission—*see* The Advisory Panel to Assess Domestic Response Capabilities for Terrorism Involving Weapons of Mass Destruction.

Hanford, D. J., "Eli Lilly: Continue to Work with FDA on Mfg Facilities," Dow Jones News Service, January 24, 2002;

Henderson, D. A., T. V. Inglesby, J. G. Bartlett, et al., "Smallpox as a Biological Weapon: Medical and Public Health Management," *Journal of the American Medical Association*, No. 281, 1999, pp. 2127–2137.

Hensley, Scott, "American Home and FDA Settle," *Wall Street Journal*, October 4, 2000, p. B8.

Inglesby, T. V., D. A. Henderson, J. G. Bartlett, et al., "Anthrax as a Biological Weapon: Medical and Public Health Management,"

Journal of the American Medical Association, No. 281, 1999, pp. 1735–1745.

Inglesby, T. V., D. T. Dennis, D. A. Henderson, et al., "Plague as a Biological Weapon," *Journal of the American Medical Association*, No. 283, 2000, pp. 2281–2290.

Japsen, B., "Abbott Laboratories Await Regulators Review of Manufacturing Processes," *Chicago Tribune*, March 6, 2002.

Javitt, G., "Drugs and Vaccines for the Common Defense: Refining FDA Regulation to Promote the Availability of Products to Counter Biological Attacks," *Journal of Contemporary Health Law and Policy*, No. 19, 2002, pp. 37–116.

Joellenbeck, L. M., L. L. Zwanziger, J. S. Durch, and B. L. Strom, eds., *The Anthrax Vaccine: Is It Safe? Does It Work?* Washington, D.C.: IOM, National Academy Press, 2002, p. 38.

Mercer Management Consulting, *Report on the United States Vaccine Industry*, prepared for the U.S. Department of Health and Human Services, June 14, 1995.

Merrill, R. A., "The Architecture of Government Regulation of Medical Products," *Virginia Law Review*, No. 82, 1996, pp. 1757–1768.

Parkman, P. D., and M. C. Hardegree, "Regulation and Testing of Vaccines," in S. A. Plotkin and W. A. Orenstein, eds., *Vaccines*, 3rd ed., Philadelphia: W. B. Saunders, 1999, pp. 1131–1143.

Petersen, M., and R. Abelson, "Drug Makers and FDA Fighting Hard Over Quality," *New York Times*, May 17, 2002, p. A1.

Pharmaceutical Research and Manufacturers of America, *Pharmaceutical Industry Profile 2001*, Washington, D.C., 2002.

Plotkin, S. A., and W. A. Orenstein, eds., *Vaccines*, 3rd ed., Philadelphia: W. B. Saunders, 1999.

Rettig, R. A., *Military Use of Drugs Not Yet Approved by FDA for CW/BW Defense: Lessons from the Gulf War*, Santa Monica, Calif.: RAND, MR-1018/9-OSD, 1999.

Rettig, R. A., *The Implementation of the Prescription Drug User Fee Act of 1992 by the Food and Drug Administration*, RAND, unpublished document.

Rettig, R. A., L. E. Earley, and R. A. Merrill, eds., *Food and Drug Administration Advisory Committees*, Washington, D.C.: IOM, National Academy Press, 1992.

Sensabaugh, S. M., "A Primer on CBER's Regulatory Review Structure and Process," *Drug Information Journal,* No. 32, 1998, pp. 1011–1030.

Stratton, K. R., J. S. Durch, and R. S. Lawrence, eds., *Vaccines for the 21st Century: A Tool for Decisionmaking*, Washington, D.C.: IOM, National Academy Press, 2000.

Strom Thurmond National Defense Authorization Act for Fiscal Year 1999, Section 731 (Public Law 105-261), October 17, 1998.

Taylor, J. M., and S. Masiello, "Team Biologics, Standard Operating Procedures for Compliance Activities," FDA memorandum, June 12, 2001.

The Advisory Panel to Assess Domestic Response Capabilities for Terrorism Involving Weapons of Mass Destruction (Gilmore Commission), *Third Annual Report to the President and the Congress,* December 15, 2001.

Thurmond Act—*see* Strom Thurmond National Defense Authorization Act for Fiscal Year 1999.

Tufts [University] Center for the Study of Drug Development, "Tufts Center for the Study of Drug Development Pegs Cost of a New Prescription Medicine at $802 Million," press release, November 30, 2001.

U.S. Department of Defense, Acquisition of Vaccine Production, *Report to the Deputy Secretary of Defense by the Independent Panel of Experts, Vol. I,* December 2000 [This document is included in DoD (2001a).]

U.S. Department of Defense, *Report on Biological Warfare Defense Vaccine Research & Development Programs*, July 2001a.

U.S. Department of Defense, Chemical and Biological Defense Program, *Annual Report to Congress and Performance Plan,* July 2001b.

U.S. Food and Drug Administration, "Vaccine Product Approval Process," July 27, 2001, available at www.fda.gov/cber/vaccine/vacappr.htm (accessed July 2003).

U.S. Food and Drug Administration, "FDA Approves License Supplements for Anthrax Vaccine: Lots from Renovated Facility Can Be Released and Distributed," press release (*FDA News*), January 31, 2002a, available at www.fda.gov/bbs/topics/NEWS/2002/NEW00792.html (accessed July 2003).

U.S. Food and Drug Administration, "Team Biologics: A Plan for Reinventing FDA's Ability to Optimize Compliance of Regulated Biologics Industries," April 12, 2002b, available at www.fda.gov/cber/genadmin/teambio.htm (accessed July 2003).

U.S. Food and Drug Administration, "FDA Approves Pyridostigmine Bromide as a Pretreatment Against Nerve Gas," press release (*FDA News*), February 5, 2003a, available at www.fda.gov/bbs/topics/NEWS/2003/NEW00870.html (accessed August 2003).

U.S. Food and Drug Administration, *Investigations Operations Manual 2003*, 2003b, available at www.fda.gov/ora/inspect_ref/iom/default.htm (accessed July 2003).

U.S. Food and Drug Administration, Center for Drug Evaluation and Research, "NDAs Approved in Calendar Years 1990–2002 by Therapeutic Potentials and Chemical Types," table, January 14, 2003, available at www.fda.gov/cder/rdmt/pstable.htm (accessed July 2003).

U.S. Food and Drug Administration, Team Biologics, *Standard Operating Procedures: Core Team Responsibilities and Procedures,* n.d.

Weiss, R., "Bioterrorism: An Even More Devastating Threat," *Washington Post,* September 17, 2001, p. A24.

Wyeth, *Wyeth GMP Systems Manual: Level II Guideline,* Training Document No. GDL 3-1-1P, July 4, 2001.

Zoon, K. C., Director, CBER, statement before the Subcommittee on National Security, Veterans Affairs, and International Relations, Committee on Government Reform, U.S. House of Representatives, April 29, 1999, at www.fda.gov/ola/1999/anthraxvaccine.html (accessed July 2003).

ABOUT THE AUTHORS

Richard A. Rettig, senior social scientist, has been at RAND from 1995 to the present and previously from 1975 until 1981. He is author of *Military Use of Drugs Not Yet Approved by FDA for CW/BW Defense: Lessons from the Gulf War* (RAND, MR-1018/9-OSD, 1999) and served as principal organizer of a RAND workshop, "FDA and the Common Defense," held in Arlington, Virginia, on December 19, 2002. Rettig also served on the professional staff of the Institute of Medicine from 1987 until 1995. While there, he directed a study of FDA advisory committees (Rettig, Earley, and Merrill, 1992).

Jennifer Brower, full engineer, has been at RAND since 1997. Her research focuses on the U.S. national security and policy implications of emerging technologies and evolving asymmetric threats. Brower is codirector of RAND's support to the congressionally mandated Advisory Panel to Assess Domestic Response Capabilities for Terrorism Involving Weapons of Mass Destruction (Gilmore Commission). She recently coauthored *The Global Threat of New and Reemerging Infectious Diseases: Reconciling U.S. National Security and Public Health Policy* (RAND, MR-1602-RC, 2003) and has published work on a smallpox vaccination policy model in the *New England Journal of Medicine.* Brower serves as an adjunct professor at George Washington University, where she recently taught a course on chemical and biological terrorism and warfare.